SOAP
for
Urology

Check out the entire SOAP series!

SOAP for Cardiology

SOAP for Emergency Medicine

SOAP for Family Medicine

SOAP for Internal Medicine

SOAP for Obstetrics and Gynecology

SOAP for Neurology

SOAP for Orthopedics

SOAP for Pediatrics

SOAP for Urology

SOAP
for
Urology

Stanley Zaslau, MD, FACS

Associate Professor

Division of Urology, Department of Surgery

West Virginia University

Morgantown, WV

Series Editor

Peter S. Uzelac, MD, FACOG

Assistant Professor

Department of Obstetrics and Gynecology

University of Southern California Keck School of Medicine

Los Angeles, California

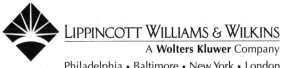

LIPPINCOTT WILLIAMS & WILKINS

A **Wolters Kluwer** Company

Philadelphia • Baltimore • New York • London
Buenos Aires • Hong Kong • Sydney • Tokyo

Acquisitions Editor: Beverly Copland
Development Editor: Selene Steneck
Production Editor: Jennifer Kowalewski
Interior and Cover Designer: Meral Dabcovich
Compositor: International Typesetting and Composition in India
Printer: Sheridan Books in Ann Arbor, MI

351 West Camden Street

Baltimore, MD 21201

530 Walnut Street
Philadelphia, PA 19106

Library of Congress Cataloging-in-Publication Data

Zaslau, Stanley.

    SOAP for urology / Stanley Zaslau.
       p. ; cm. — (SOAP series)
    Includes index.
    ISBN-13: 978-1-4051-0451-7 (pbk. : alk. paper)
    ISBN-10: 1-4051-0451-1 (pbk. : alk. paper) 1. Urology—Handbooks, manuals, etc.
    [DNLM: 1. Urogenital Diseases—Handbooks. 2. Urologic Diseases—Handbooks.
    WJ 39 Z385 2006] I. Title: Urology. II. Title. III. Series.
    RC872.9.Z39 2006
    616.6—dc22

                                      2005010320

To purchase additional copies of this book, call our customer service department at **(800) 638-3030** or fax orders to **(301) 824-7390**. International customers should call **(301) 714-2324**.

Visit Lippincott Williams & Wilkins on the Internet: http://www.LWW.com.
Lippincott Williams & Wilkins customer service representatives are available from 8:30 am to 6:00 pm, EST.

05 06 07 08 09
1 2 3 4 5 6 7 8 9 10

Contents

Contributors

Brian DeFade, DO
Resident, Surgery
Charleston Area Medical Center
Charleston, West Virginia

John C. Lynam
Medical Student IV
Western University/College of Osteopathic Medicine of the Pacific
Pomona, California

Michael Mastromichalis, MD
Resident, Surgery
University of Virginia School of Medicine
Charlottesville, Virginia

Jonathan Mobley, MD
Resident, Urology
West Virginia University School of Medicine
Morgantown, West Virginia

Justin Nelms, MD
Resident, Surgery
Allegheny General Hospital
Pittsburgh, Pennsylvania

Adam E. Perlmutter, DO
Resident, Urology
West Virginia University School of Medicine
Morgantown, West Virginia

Stephen Sparks, MD
Resident, Urology
West Virginia University School of Medicine
Morgantown, West Virginia

Reviewers

Amir A. Ghaferi
4th year student
Johns Hopkins University School of Medicine
Baltimore, Maryland

Gina Murrary
4th year student
The Brody School of Medicine at East Carolina University
Greenville, North Carolina

Sarah K. Taylor, MD
Resident
Children's Hospital & Regional Medical Center/University of Washington
Seattle, Washington

Randall Young
4th year student
UC Davis School of Medicine
Davis, California

To the Reader

Like most medical students, I started my ward experience head down and running, eager to finally make contact with real patients. What I found was a confusing world, completely different from anything I had known during the first two years of medical school. New language, foreign abbreviations and residents too busy to set my bearings straight: Where would I begin?

Pocket textbooks, offering medical knowledge in a convenient and portable package, seemed to be the logical solution. Unfortunately, I found myself spending valuable time sifting through large amounts of text, often not finding the answer to my question, and in the process, missing out on teaching points during rounds!

I designed the SOAP series to provide medical students and house staff with pocket manuals that truly serve their intended purpose: quick accessibility to the most practical clinical information in a user-friendly format. At the inception of this project, I envisioned all of the benefits the SOAP format would bring to the reader:

- Learning through this model reinforces a thought process that is already familiar to students and residents, facilitating easier long-term retention.

- SOAP promotes good communication between physicians and facilitates the teaching/learning process.

- SOAP puts the emphasis back on the patient's clinical problem and not the diagnosis.

- In the age of managed care, SOAP meets the challenge of providing efficiency while maintaining quality.

- As sound medical-legal practice gains attention in physician training, SOAP emphasizes adherence to a documentation style that leaves little room for potential misinterpretation.

Rather than attempting to summarize the contents of a thousand-page textbook into a miniature form, the SOAP series focuses exclusively on guidance through patient encounters. In a typical use, "finding out where to start" or "refreshing your memory" with SOAP books should be possible in less than a minute. Subjects are always confined to two pages and the most important points have been highlighted. Topics have been limited to those problems you will most commonly encounter repeatedly during your training and contents are grouped according to the hospital or clinic setting. Facts and figures that are not particularly helpful to surviving life on the wards, such as demographics, pathophysiology and busy tables and graphs have purposely been omitted (such details are much better studied in a quiet environment using large and comprehensive texts).

Congratulations on your achievements thus far and I wish you a highly successful medical career!

Peter S. Uzelac, MD, FACOG

Acknowledgments

Thanks to Dr. Pete Uzelac for allowing *SOAP for Urology* to be a part of his very successful SOAP notes series. Selene Steneck has done another outstanding job as my editor. Special thanks to Bev Copland for her continued support of my work. Finally, thanks to my WVU urology residents and students who fuel my passion to be their teacher.

Stanley Zaslau, MD, FACS

Abbreviations

ABG	arterial blood gas
ACE	angiotensin-converting enzyme
AFP	alpha-fetoprotein
AIDS	acquired immunodeficiency syndrome
BP	blood pressure
BPH	benign prostatic hyperplasia
BUN	blood urea nitrogen
CAH	congenital adrenal hyperplasia
CBC	complete blood count
CIS	carcinoma in situ
CT	computed tomography
CXR	chest x-ray
DLPP	detrusor leak point pressure
DRE	digital rectal examination
ECG	electrocardiograph
hCG	human chorionic gonadotropin
HIV	human immunodeficiency virus
HPV	human papillomavirus
HVA	homovanillic acid
ICU	intensive care unit
IM	intramuscular
IPSS	International Prostate Symptom Score
IV	intravenous
LDH	lactate dehydrogenase
min	minute
MRI	magnetic resonance imaging
NSAIDs	nonsteroidal anti-inflammatory drugs
PA	posteroanterior
PLAP	placental alkaline phosphatase
PO	by mouth
PRN	as needed
PSA	prostate-specific antigen
PUV	posterior urethral valve
RBC	red blood cells
RCC	renal cell carcinoma
SSRI	selective serotonin reuptake inhibitors
STAT	immediately
SUI	sudden urge incontinence
TID	three times daily
TMP/SMX	trimethoprim/sulfamethoxazole
UA	urinalysis
UPJ	ureteropelvic junction
VCUG	voiding cystourethrogram
VHL	von Hippel-Lindau disease
VLPP	Valsalva leak point pressure
VMA	vanillylmandelic acid
VUR	vesicoureteral reflux
WBC	white blood cell
wk(s)	week(s)
yr(s)	year(s)

Normal Lab Values

Blood, Plasma, Serum

Aminotransferase, alanine (ALT, SGPT)	0–35 U/L
Aminotransferase, aspartate (AST, SGOT)	0–35 U/L
Ammonia, plasma	40–80 µg/dL
Amylase, serum	0–130 U/L
Antistreptolysin O titer	Less than 150 units
Bicarbonate, serum	23–28 meq/L
Bilirubin, serum	
Total	0.3–1.2 mg/dL
Direct	0–0.3 mg/dL
Blood gases, arterial (room air)	
P_{O_2}	80–100 mm Hg
P_{CO_2}	35–45 mm Hg
pH	7.38–7.44
Calcium, serum	9–10.5 mg/dL
Carbon dioxide content, serum	23–28 meq/L
Chloride, serum	98–106 meq/L
Cholesterol, total, plasma	150–199 mg/dL (desirable)
Cholesterol, low-density lipoprotein (LDL), plasma	≤130 mg/dL (desirable)
Cholesterol, high-density lipoprotein (HDL), plasma	≥40 mg/dL (desirable)
Complement, serum	
C3	55–120 mg/dL
Total	37–55 U/mL
Copper, serum	70–155 µg/dL
Creatine kinase, serum	30–170 U/L
Creatinine, serum	0.7–1.3 mg/dL
Ethanol, blood	<50 mg/dL
Fibrinogen, plasma	150–350 mg/dL
Folate, red cell	160–855 ng/mL
Folate, serum	2.5–20 ng/mL
Glucose, plasma	
Fasting	70–105 mg/dL
2 hours postprandial	<140 mg/dL
Iron, serum	60–160 µg/dL
Iron binding capacity, serum	250–460 µg/dL
Lactate dehydrogenase, serum	60–100 U/L
Lactic acid, venous blood	6–16 mg/dL
Lead, blood	<40 µg/dL

Lipase, serum	<95 U/L
Magnesium, serum	1.5–2.4 mg/dL
Manganese, serum	0.3–0.9 ng/mL
Methylmalonic acid, serum	150–370 nmol/L
Osmolality plasma	275–295 mOsm/kg H_2O
Phosphatase, acid, serum	0.5–5.5 U/L
Phosphatase, alkaline, serum	36–92 U/L
Phosphorus, inorganic, serum	3–4.5 mg/dL
Potassium, serum	3.5–5 meq/L
Protein, serum	
Total	6.0–7.8 g/dL
Albumin	3.5–5.5 g/dL
Globulins	2.5–3.5 g/dL
$Alpha_1$	0.2–0.4 g/dL
$Alpha_2$	0.5–0.9 g/dL
Beta	0.6–1.1 g/dL
Gamma	0.7–1.7 g/dL
Rheumatoid factor	<40 U/mL
Sodium, serum	136–145 meq/L
Triglycerides	<250 mg/dL (desirable)
Urea nitrogen, serum	8–20 mg/dL
Uric acid, serum	2.5–8 mg/dL
Vitamin B_{12}, serum	200–800 pg/mL

Cerebrospinal Fluid

Cell count	0–5 cells/μL
Glucose (less than 40% of simultaneous plasma concentration is abnormal)	40–80 mg/dL
Protein	15–60 mg/dL
Pressure (opening)	70–200 cm H_2O

Endocrine

Adrenocorticotropin (ACTH)	9–52 pg/mL
Aldosterone, serum	
Supine	2–5 ng/dL
Standing	7–20 ng/dL
Aldosterone, urine	5–19 μg/24 h
Cortisol	
Serum 8 AM	8–20 μg/dL
5 PM	3–13 μg/dL
1 h after cosyntropin	>18 μg/dL
usually ≥8 μg/dL above baseline	

overnight suppression test	<5 μg/dL
Urine free cortisol	<90 μg/24 h
Estradiol, serum	
Male	10–30 pg/mL
Female	
Cycle day 1–10	50–100 pmol/L
Cycle day 11–20	50–200 pmol/L
Cycle day 21–30	70–150 pmol/L
Estriol, urine	>12 mg/24 h
Follicle-stimulating hormone, serum	
Male (adult)	5–15 mU/mL
Female	
Follicular or luteal phase	5–20 mU/mL
Midcycle peak	30–50 mU/mL
Postmenopausal	>35 mU/mL
Insulin, serum (fasting)	5–20 mU/L
17-ketosteroids, urine	
Male	8–22 mg/24 h
Female	Up to 15 μg/24 h
Luteinizing hormone, serum	
Male	3–15 mU/mL (3–15 U/L)
Female	
Follicular or luteal phase	5–22 mU/mL
Midcycle peak	30–250 mU/mL
Postmenopausal	>30 mU/mL
Parathyroid hormone, serum	10–65 pg/mL
Progesterone	
Luteal	3–30 ng/mL
Follicular	<1 ng/mL
Prolactin, serum	
Male	<15 ng/mL
Female	<20 ng/mL
Testosterone, serum	
Adult male	300–1200 ng/dL
Female	20–75 ng/dL
Thyroid function tests (normal ranges vary)	
Thyroid iodine (^{131}I) uptake	10% to 30% of administered dose at 24 h
Thyroid-stimulating hormone (TSH)	0.5–5.0 μU/mL
Thyroxine (T4), serum	
Total	5–12 pg/dL
Free	0.9–2.4 ng/dL

Free T4 index   4–11
Triiodothyronine, resin (T3)   25%–35%
Triiodothyronine, serum (T3)   70–195 ng/dL
Vitamin D
   1,25-dihydroxy, serum   25–65 pg/mL
   25-hydroxy, serum   15–80 ng/mL

Gastrointestinal

Fecal urobilinogen   40–280 mg/24 h
Gastrin, serum   0–180 pg/mL
Lactose tolerance test
   Increase in plasma glucose   >15 mg/dL
Lipase, ascitic fluid   <200 U/L
Secretin-cholecystokinin pancreatic function   >80 meq/L of HCO_3 in at least
          1 specimen collected over 1 h
Stool fat   <5 g/d on a 100-g fat diet
Stool nitrogen   <2 g/d
Stool weight   <200 g/d

Hematology

Activated partial thromboplastin time   25–35 s
Bleeding time   <10 min
Coagulation factors, plasma
   Factor I   150–350 mg/dL
   Factor II   60%–150% of normal
   Factor V   60%–150% of normal
   Factor VII   60%–150% of normal
   Factor VIII   60%–150% of normal
   Factor IX   60%–150% of normal
   Factor X   60%–150% of normal
   Factor XI   60%–150% of normal
   Factor XII   60%–150% of normal
Erythrocyte count   4.2–5.9 million cells/μL
Erythropoietin   <30 mU/mL
D-dimer   <0.5 μg/mL
Ferritin, serum   15–200 ng/mL
Glucose-6-phosphate dehydrogenase, blood   5–15 U/g Hgb
Haptoglobin, serum   50–150 mg/dL
Hematocrit
   Male   41%–51%
   Female   36%–47%

Hemoglobin, blood	
Male	14–17 g/dL
Female	12–16 g/dL
Hemoglobin, plasma	0.5–5 mg/dL
Leukocyte alkaline phosphatase	15–40 mg of phosphorus liberated/h per 10^{10} cells
Score	13–130/100 polymorphonuclear neutrophils and band forms
Leukocyte count	
Nonblacks	4000–10,000/µL
Blacks	3500–10,000/µL
Lymphocytes	
CD4+ cell count	640–1175/µL
CD8+ cell count	335–875/µL
CD4:CD8 ratio	1.0–4.0
Mean corpuscular hemoglobin (MCH)	28–32 pg
Mean corpuscular hemoglobin concentration (MCHC)	32–36 g/dL
Mean corpuscular volume (MCV)	80–100 fL
Platelet count	150,000–350,000/µL
Protein C activity, plasma	67%–I 31%
Protein C resistance	2.2–2.6
Protein S activity, plasma	82%–144%
Prothrombin time	11–13 s
Reticulocyte count	0.5%–1.5% of erythrocytes
Absolute	23,000–90,000 cells/µL
Schilling test (oral administration of radioactive cobalamin-labeled vitamin B_{12})	8.5%–28% excreted in urine per 24–48 h
Sedimentation rate, erythrocyte (Westergren)	
Male	0–15 mm/h
Female	0–20 mm/h
Volume, blood	
Plasma	
Male	25–44 mL/kg body weight
Female	28–43 mL/kg body weight
Erythrocyte	
Male	25–35 mL/kg body weight
Female	20–30 mL/kg body weight

Urine

Amino acids	200–400 mg/24 h
Amylase	6.5–48.1 U/h

Calcium	100–300 mg/d on unrestricted diet
Chloride	80–250 meq/d (varies with intake)
Copper	0–100 µg/24 h
Creatine	
Male	4–40 mg/24 h
Female	0–100 mg/24 h
Creatinine	15–25 mg/kg per 24 h
Creatinine clearance	90–140 mL/min
Osmolality	38–1400 mOsm/kg H_2O
Phosphate, tubular resorption	79%–94% (0.79–0.94) of filtered load
Potassium	25–100 meq/24 h (varies with intake)
Protein	<100 mg/24 h
Sodium	100–260 meq/24h (varies with intake)
Uric acid	250–750 mg/24 h (varies with diet)
Urobilinogen	0.05–2.5 mg/24 h

Seminal Fluid Analysis

Appearance	Opaque, gray-white, highly viscid
Volume	2–5 mL
Liquefaction	Complete within 30 min
pH	7.2–8.0
Leukocytes	Occasional or absent
Count	20–250 million/mL
Motility	50%–80% with progressive active motility
Morphology	50%–90% with normal forms

I
Genitourinary Oncology

Does the pt complain of having a testis mass?

65% to 94% of pts present with a painless, unilateral testicular mass, or swelling of one testicle that was found by either the pt or his partner.

Is the mass painless or painful?
The presenting symptom may be acute testicular pain, and in other instances the presenting symptoms may be related to metastasis: lymphadenopathy, respiratory, bone pain, and gastrointestinal complaints.

Does the pt have shortness of breath?
Pts with pulmonary metastases can present with dyspnea and shortness of breath.

Does the pt have weight loss?
Significant weight loss (>10 pounds) in the absence of dieting may suggest advanced disease.

 Perform a physical examination
Physical exam may be benign in pts with an incidentally found testis mass.
  • Incidentally found by the pt's partner or himself.
  • In more advanced disease, supraclavicular lymphadenopathy may be identified. Examine for gynecomastia, lower-extremity swelling, and lumbar back pain.
  • Palpation of the abdomen should be done to rule out any masses or nodal enlargement.

Evaluate the involved and contralateral testicle
Begin with contralateral side for baseline, and then compare to affected side.
  • Any solid/hard areas should be suspicious for neoplasm.

Obtain a scrotal sonogram
Should be performed to rule out other causes such as hydrocele, or epididymitis.
  • Any hypoechoic area in tunica albuginea is suspicious for testicular carcinoma.

Obtain serum tumor marker levels
Alpha-fetoprotein (AFP): Should not be elevated in pure seminomas.
Human chorionic gonadotropin (hCG): Elevated in 10% of pts with pure seminoma. Increased hCG levels cause gynecomastia.
Lactic acid dehydrogenase (LDH): There is a direct relationship between tumor burden and LDH levels—the higher the stage of disease, the higher the LDH level.
Placental alkaline phosphatase: Elevated in 40% of pts with advanced disease.

Obtain imaging studies
Posteroanterior (PA) and lateral CXR: to rule out lung metastasis.
CT scan: important for identifying retroperitoneal lymph node and liver involvement.

Make definitive diagnosis with inguinal exploration
Orchiectomy: definitive procedure to both diagnose and locally stage testicular cancer.

Male with unilateral testis mass

Consider differential diagnosis of testis mass

A unilateral testicular mass should always be considered a testicular tumor until proven otherwise.

Differential diagnosis

Consider: hydrocele, varicocele, spermatocele, hematocele, acute orchitis, and epididymitis. In addition, one should also consider: testicular torsion, strangulated hernia, and testicular carcinoma.

 Treatment

Treat low stage seminoma with orchiectomy and radiotherapy

Stage I seminoma: Pts with localized disease.

- The recommended treatment is orchiectomy followed by local, adjuvant radiation to retroperitoneal lymph nodes.
- These pts should be followed long term for recurrence.

Treat seminoma with bulky lymph nodes with orchiectomy and adjuvant chemotherapy

Stage IIa and IIb seminoma: Pts with bulky retroperitoneal disease. These pts receive adjuvant radiation therapy.

- For those with masses larger than 5 cm in diameter, adjuvant chemotherapy is recommended.

Treat advanced seminoma with adjuvant chemotherapy

Stage IIc and stage III—advanced seminoma:

- Cisplatin-based chemotherapy is the modality of choice, residual masses after chemotherapeutic treatment may be removed surgically.

Treat nonseminomas aggressively

Nonseminomas have a higher chance lymph node metastasis.

- Low stage tumors are treated with retroperitoneal lymphadenectomy while advanced tumors (stage II and higher) are treated first with multiagent chemotherapy.

Does the pt have a testicular mass?
Pt may find a firm, non-tender mass in both testes.
- However, the presenting symptom may be acute testicular pain.

Was the pt recently treated for epididymitis or hydrocele?
Pts with testicular carcinoma are often misdiagnosed with epididymitis, or a hydrocele.

Did this pt ever have surgery for an undescended testicle?
Pts with bilateral testicular tumors may have had orchiopexy as children because of undescended testis/cryptorchidism.

Does the pt have shortness of breath?
Pts with pulmonary metastases can present with dyspnea and shortness of breath.

Does the pt have weight loss?
Significant weight loss (>10 pounds) in the absence of dieting may suggest advanced disease.

Perform a physical examination
Physical exam may be benign in pts with a testicular mass.
- In more advanced disease, supraclavicular lymphadenopathy may be identified. Gynecomastia, lower-extremity swelling, and lumbar back pain may be found.
- Palpation of the abdomen should be done to rule out any masses or nodal enlargement.

Evaluate both testicles carefully for masses
Begin with contralateral side for baseline, and then compare to affected side.
- Any solid/hard areas should be suspicious for neoplasm.

Perform scrotal ultrasound
Should be done to rule out other causes: hydrocele, or epididymitis. Any hypoechoic area in tunica albuginea is suspicious for testicular carcinoma.

Obtain blood for serum tumor markers
Alpha-fetoprotein (AFP): Should not be elevated in pure seminomas.
Human chorionic gonadotropin (hCG): Usually increased 10% of pts with pure seminoma. Increased hCG levels cause gynecomastia.
Lactic acid dehydrogenase (LDH): There is a direct relationship between tumor burden and LDH levels—the higher the stage of disease, the higher the LDH level.
Placental alkaline phosphatase: elevated in 40% of pts with advanced disease.
Prostate-specific antigen: metastasis from prostate carcinoma accounts for 75% of bilateral testicular masses.

Obtain imaging studies
Posteroanterior and lateral CXR: used to rule out lung metastasis.
CT scan: good for identifying liver and retroperitoneal lymph node involvement.

Male with bilateral testis mass

Consider differential diagnosis of testis tumors: Bold font = increased incidence of bilateral tumors
Germ cell tumors (95%)
    Seminoma 50%
    Spermatocytic seminoma
    Embryonal carcinoma 20%
    Teratocarcinoma 10%
    Teratoma 5%
Gonadal stromal tumors (5%)
    Leydig cell tumors 5%
    Sertoli cell tumor
Metastatic tumors
    Leukemia
    Lymphoma
    Melanoma
    Prostate
    Lung

 Treatment

Consider prior medical history before treatment plan

Pts with bilateral testis masses are more likely to have a history of cryptorchidism/undescended testis.

- 1% to 2% of testicular tumors are bilateral, and 50% of those are associated with cryptorchidism.
- Seminoma is the most common primary tumor.

Consider presence of systemic syndromes associated with bilateral testis masses

Some syndromes have been shown to have an increased incidence of bilateral testicular masses. Carney's complex and adrenogenital syndrome are two examples.

Consider treatment for localized seminoma
Stage I seminoma: Orchiectomy followed by local, adjuvant radiation to retroperitoneal lymph nodes. These pts should be observed long term for recurrence.

Consider alternative treatments for seminoma with bulky lymph nodes
Stage IIa and IIb seminoma: Pts with bulky retroperitoneal disease. These pts receive adjuvant radiation therapy. For those with masses larger than 5 cm in diameter, adjuvant chemotherapy is preferred.

Consider adjuvant chemotherapy for advanced seminoma
Stage IIc and stage III—advanced seminoma: These pts have bulky retroperitoneal disease above the diaphragm. Cisplatin-based chemotherapy seems to be the modality of choice. Residual masses after chemotherapeutic treatment has ceased may be removed surgically.

Treat nonseminomatous germ cell tumors aggressively
Nonseminomas have a higher chance of metastasis to the lymph nodes.
- Low stage tumors are treated with retroperitoneal lymph node dissection, while advanced tumors (stage II and higher) are treated first with multiagent chemotherapy.

S **Does this pt have irritative or obstructive voiding symptoms?**

Irritative or obstructive voiding symptoms are common with benign prostatic
hypertrophy (BPH)

- Obstructive symptoms include incomplete emptying, hesitancy, weak urinary
  stream, dribbling, and straining to urinate.
- Irritative symptoms include urinary urgency, nocturia, incontinence, and
  frequency.
- Urinary retention, urinary tract infections, and hematuria are other symptoms
  noted.

Does this pt have perineal pain, back pain, or dysuria?

Perineal pain, back pain, and dysuria suggest prostatitis

Because prostatitis can be either acute or chronic, the presenting symptoms vary.
- **Acute:** there is usually abrupt onset of fever, chills, myalgias, lower back pain,
  perineal pain, and rectal pain.
- Urinary symptoms include terminal dysuria, urgency, frequency, and pain with
  ejaculation.
- **Chronic:** has more insidious onset including recurrent urinary tract infections
  (UTI). Some complain of dysuria, frequency, nocturia, perineal pain, and low
  back pain.

Does the pt have any symptoms to suggest prostate cancer?
Pts with prostate cancer are usually asymptomatic, although they may present with
weight loss, and obstructive/irritative voiding symptoms.
- Bone pain, lymphedema, fecal incontinence, and urinary incontinence from
  metastasis are other symptoms that should be addressed.

 Perform a physical examination

A digital rectal exam (DRE), urinalysis (UA), and a prostate-specific antigen (PSA)
level are three tests to differentiate which entity is causing the elevation of PSA.

Perform a digital rectal examination

Is the prostate symmetrically enlarged?
In BPH, the prostate may be symmetrically enlarged.
- The PSA increases 0.12 ng/mL per gram of prostate tissue.

Is the prostate tender and boggy?
In prostatitis, the DRE reveals an enlarged, tender, boggy prostate.
- The UA will show bacteriuria, and increased white blood cells.
- Positive expressed prostate secretions indicate prostatic infection. The PSA may
  be elevated.

Is a palpable nodule present?
In prostate cancer, the DRE reveals an enlarged, nodular, irregular prostate.

- Not all pts with prostate cancer will have an abnormal DRE.

Obtain serum PSA

A PSA level above 4.0 ng/mL (or above age-specific levels) in the absence of infection
or an abnormal DRE suggests prostate cancer and requires prostate needle biopsy.

PSA will increase by greater than 0.75 ng/mL per year in pts with prostate cancer.

Obtain additional laboratory tests
Serum creatinine: should be drawn in all pts to rule out obstructive uropathy.

Consider prostate needle biopsy
Transrectal ultrasound-guided needle biopsy: Any pt with a positive DRE or an
elevated PSA should undergo prostate needle biopsy.

Obtain imaging studies
Bone scan and CXR: Should be performed in those pts suspected of having prostate
carcinoma with positive back pain to rule out distant metastasis.

Obtain American Urological Association (AUA)/IPSS score
A seven-item questionnaire to assess pt's voiding symptoms. Scored on a scale of 0 to
35. Scores of 0 to 7 suggest mild symptoms, 8 to 19 suggest moderate symptoms,
and scores above 20 suggest severe symptoms.
  • AUA/IPSS symptom score should be obtained in pts with voiding complaints.

Consider urodynamic evaluation
Pressure flow studies, and residual urine volume determination: Can be used to
assess the degree of obstruction in pts with BPH.

Elevated PSA

Differential diagnosis
Elevated PSA can be due to prostate cancer. Prostate biopsy must be considered.
Other causes of elevated PSA include prostatitis, recent prostate needle biopsy, recent
cystoscopy, recent or current urinary catheterization.

Consider pharmacotherapy

**Pharmacotherapy is used for pts with symptomatic benign
prostatic hypertrophy (BPH).**
Use 5-alpha reductase inhibitors (5ARIs) such as finasteride and dutasteride, and
alpha-receptor blockers (tamsulosin, terazosin, and doxazosin) for mild-to-moderate
symptoms.
  • Alpha blockers considered first-line treatment for BPH.
  • 5ARI recommended in pts with PSA > 1.5 mg/mL and/or prostate size greater
    than 30 g.

Consider surgical therapy
Particularly in pts with moderate-to-severe symptoms.
  • Options include transurethral resection of prostate (TURP), microwave ther-
    motherapy, lasers, high-temperature radio frequency ablation of prostate, high
    intensity ultrasound, and open prostatectomy.

Consider watchful waiting
A majority of pts will respond to simple follow-up surveillance. Treatment can be
modified at follow-up visits.

Initiate antibiotic therapy for prostatitis
Acute prostatitis: treatment is with antibiotic therapy—trimethoprim/sulfamethoxa-
zole, or a quinolone is recommended for 4 to 6 weeks of therapy.
Chronic prostatitis: treated with antibiotic therapy, but for a longer duration—3 to
4 months.

Consider treatments for prostate cancer
Treatment will vary with pt's age and general health status.
May include radical prostatectomy, brachytherapy, external beam radiotherapy,
cryotherapy, hormonal therapy, or watchful waiting.

S

How was this pt treated for prostate cancer?
It would be important to obtain this information to begin assessment.
- Determine mode of previous treatment
  - Radical prostatectomy
  - Brachytherapy
  - Orchiectomy
  - Observation
  - External beam radiotherapy
  - Cryotherapy
  - Hormonal therapy

When was the last treatment and what was the nadir prostate-specific antigen?
An early increase in prostate-specific antigen (PSA) after treatment is a poor prognostic sign.

If the pt had radical prostatectomy, what were the pathologic findings?

Cancer recurrence after radical prostatectomy is related to cancer grade, pathologic stage, and the degree of extracapsular extension.
- Cancer recurrence is more common in those pts with positive surgical margins, established extracapsular extension, seminal vesicle invasion, and high-grade disease.

What is the pt's PSA?

After radical prostatectomy, the PSA should be zero, and remain undetectable.
- Pts whose PSA becomes detectable early after treatment and those with PSA levels that double rapidly are more likely to have systemic relapse.

O

Perform a physical examination

Evaluate the prostate fossa for masses
Physical exam in these pts is often negative.
- Occasionally there may be palpable induration on digital rectal examination (DRE) of the prostatic fossa.
- Pts with recurrent disease and distant metastasis may have back pain, fatigue, or weight loss.

Obtain a serum PSA
PSA may be elevated. PSA doubling at three consecutive draws (6 months apart) suggests recurrence.

Perform CT and bone scan
CT should be performed to evaluate metastasis to the lung, liver, and lymph nodes. Bone scan will evaluate for skeletal metastasis.

Consider ProstaScint scan
Radioimmunoscintigraphy: approved by the US Food and Drug Administration (FDA) for evaluating pts with increasing PSA levels post-prostatectomy.

Prostate cancer with increase in PSA after treatment
Prostate cancer with an increase in PSA is seen in about 5% of pts at 5 years after prostatectomy who have confined prostate gland disease.
- This percentage doubles to about 11% in pts with prostate capsular penetration. Seminal vesicle involvement increases the percentage to 66%, and lymphatic involvement increases the chance of the PSA increasing post-prostatectomy to 76%.

Gleason score and the PSA doubling time become an important indicator of whether the disease has local or distant recurrence, and can be a measure of treatment options.

Consider surveillance protocol
Pts should be followed with serum PSA levels every 3 months after prostatectomy has been performed for the first year. For the next 4 years, the pts' PSA should be followed every 6 months, and every year thereafter.
In pts who the PSA serially increases for 2 consecutive follow-up visits, additional treatment and evaluation are warranted.

Consider parameters for treatment
Treatment options are determined by several factors such as local vs. distant recurrence, Gleason score, age, and PSA doubling time.

Consider radiation therapy for pts with local recurrence
These pts tend to have low Gleason scores, and long PSA doubling times after prostatectomy. These pts should be treated with radiation first.
- Androgen ablation should be considered in pts who fail radiation treatment.

Consider androgen ablation treatment for pts with distant metastases
These pts tend to have higher post-prostatectomy Gleason scores, and much shorter PSA doubling times.
- Androgen ablation therapy is the treatment of choice in these pts. This therapy can be accomplished by using gonadotropin-releasing hormone agonists (leuprolide, goserelin, nafarelin, and histrelin), 5-alpha-dihydrotestosterone receptor blockade (flutamide and bicalutamide), ketoconazole, and by performing a bilateral orchiectomy.
- Radiation therapy is considered if androgen ablation fails.
- Chemotherapy is considered for hormone refractory disease.

Consider salvage radical prostatectomy
These are pts who have not had radical prostate surgery.
- The recommended treatment for these pts, if they have distant metastasis, is androgen ablation therapy. For local disease, a salvage radical prostatectomy can be considered.

Consider watchful waiting
In older pts who are in poor health, watchful waiting or androgen ablation should be considered.
- In pts who have greater than 10 years of life expectancy, radiation therapy should be considered first, followed by androgen ablation for radiation failures.

Does the pt have irritative or obstructive voiding symptoms?
Pts with early bladder carcinoma are often asymptomatic.
- Symptomatic pts present with gross hematuria 85% to 90% of the time.
- Other symptoms include frequency, urgency, dysuria, microscopic hematuria, and anemia.

Does the pt have back or flank pain?
Pts with advanced disease may have back or flank pain from metastasis.

Has the pt had any recent laboratory studies?
Pts with ureteral obstruction may present with azotemia.

Does the pt have a history of smoking?
Smoking increases a pt's risk for developing bladder cancer.
- Cigarette smoking accounts for 25% to 60% of cases of bladder cancer.

What is the pt's occupation?
Pts working in the rubber, dye, and chemical industries have an increased risk of developing bladder cancer due to exposure to beta-naphthaline and aniline dyes.

Has the pt ever had chemotherapy or radiotherapy?
Cyclophosphamide and thiotepa can be associated with hemorrhagic cystitis.

Perform a physical examination

Palpate the abdomen for abdominal masses
Physical exam may be normal. Those pts who have symptoms may present with a palpable suprapubic mass, or a rectal mass on digital rectal examination (DRE) from tumor extension to rectum.
- Hepatomegaly, supraclavicular lymphadenopathy, and lymphedema may be identified.

Perform urinalysis
Should be performed in any pt complaining of voiding symptoms or gross hematuria.

Perform urine cytology
Cells for microscopic examination are collected from voided urine.
- Urine cytology is 30% sensitive in diagnosing low-grade bladder cancer, but is excellent for detecting carcinoma in situ and high-grade lesions (90%).

Perform diagnostic cystoscopy with biopsies
This procedure can be used for diagnosis and staging of bladder cancer.

Perform intravenous pyelography
Intravenous pyelography (IVP) can detect a filling defect in the bladder 60% of the time.
- Small tumors rarely detected with IVP.
- Ideally should be obtained before transurethral resection.

Perform contrast-enhanced CT
Very useful in clinical staging of pts with advanced bladder carcinoma.
- May demonstrate thickening of the bladder wall, extravesical extension, nodal involvement or distant metastasis.

Consider metastatic workup
Consists of chest x-ray and bone scan.
- Chest x-ray is the initial screening for pulmonary metastasis.
- Bone scan is obtained in pts with invasive or locally advanced tumors and skeletal symptoms or elevated serum alkaline phosphatase.

Hematuria secondary to bladder carcinoma

Description

Pts at high risk include those who smoke, have chronic bladder infections, calculous disease, occupational exposure to chemicals (aniline dye, rubber, petroleum), previous schistosomiasis infection, and previous treatment of metastatic disease with cyclophosphamide.

Differential diagnosis

Classify tumor according to cystoscopy and biopsy results.

- Transitional cell carcinoma (90%)
  - ◆ Carcinoma in situ
- Squamous cell carcinoma (7%)
- Adenocarcinoma (2%)
- Small cell carcinoma (<1%)
- Sarcoma (<1%)
- Melanoma (<1%)

 Consider transurethral resection based on pathologic results

Superficial bladder carcinoma: treatment is transurethral resection of bladder tumor (TURBT).

- **Low-grade tumors:** treatment is complete TURBT and surveillance.
- **High-grade or recurrent bladder cancer:** treatment is complete TURBT followed by intravesical therapy (BCG, mitomycin, thiotepa).

Consider radical cystectomy for invasive disease

Invasive, but localized disease (T2-T3): treatment may include partial or radical cystectomy, radiation therapy with chemotherapy, or surgery with chemotherapy.

Invasion of adjacent tissue (T4, N+, or M+): pts are treated with systemic chemotherapy followed by either surgery or radiation therapy.

Consider prognostic factors in superficial bladder cancer

Cystoscopic finding

Tumor size	>5 cm	35% muscle invasion
	<5 cm	10% muscle invasion
Tumor number	<1 lesion	20%–60% recurrence rate
	>1 lesion	40%–90% recurrence rate

Plan follow-up care

The pt should be observed with cystoscopy every 3 months for 2 years, every 6 months for 2 more years, and annually thereafter provided that no recurrences are noted.

S **Is the pt having irritative voiding symptoms?**
Carcinoma in situ (CIS) may be asymptomatic or produce irritative voiding symptoms (urgency, frequency, bladder pain).

Does the pt have neurogenic bladder or prostatitis?
Benign prostatic enlargement, chronic prostatitis, interstitial cystitis, and neurogenic bladder can also present with irritative symptoms.

Does the pt have a history of smoking?
Smoking increases a pt's risk for developing bladder cancer.
- Cigarette smoking accounts for 25% to 60% of cases of bladder cancer.

Does the pt have symptoms of a urinary tract infection?
Approximately 30% of pts present with dysuria and irritative voiding symptoms.
- Urinalysis may reveal a urinary tract infection in 30% of pts.

 Perform a physical examination

Perform bimanual examination
Bimanual exam under anesthesia to look for fixation of the bladder to the pelvic side wall.

Perform diagnostic cystoscopy
Diagnostic cystoscopy with tumor biopsy or resection will provide information about the degree of tumor differentiation and the depth of tumor invasion.

Perform imaging studies of the upper urinary tract
Upper tract imaging studies should also be performed, which can include intravenous pyelography or CT scan of the abdomen or pelvis.

Obtain urine cytology
Urine cytology is usually positive in the presence of CIS because tumor cells slough off into the urine.

Consider MRI
MRI cannot help distinguish depth of tumor invasion. CT would be a better choice because it can determine tumor extent and the presence of enlarged lymph nodes.

Carcinoma in situ of the bladder

Symptomatic CIS

Symptomatic CIS is due to involvement of the urothelium. CIS can be found focally or in association with other papillary tumors.

Definition

CIS is defined by four characteristics: flat, erythematous, multifocal, and high grade.
- The presence of CIS is an indicator of increased biologic aggressiveness.
- Papillary or sessile tumors are more likely to recur or invade when associated with CIS.

Treatment

Consider intravesical chemotherapy

BCG is the most effective agent for most pts with CIS. It has a 70% objective response rate.
- Treatment of refractory CIS can include repeat treatment with BCG, however, some pts will require cystectomy.

Consider rationale for Bacillus of Calmette-Guérin (BCG) immunotherapy

Prevent or reduce the rate of recurrence, prevent muscle invasion of tumor cells, and to eradicate established tumor.

Method of BCG administration
1. Catheterize pt's bladder with 16F Foley catheter.
2. Mix BCG with 60 cc of saline and instill into bladder by gravity drainage.
3. Retain in bladder for approximately 90 minutes.
4. Remove Foley catheter after administration.
5. Treat weekly for 6 weeks.
6. For the second course of treatment, include maintenance therapy (3 weekly instillations every 3 months for 1 year).

Discuss side effects of BCG immunotherapy with all pts

Bladder irritative symptoms such as urinary frequency or urgency are common.
- Some pts can develop mild systemic symptoms such as development of a low-grade fever and myalgias.
- Persistently high fevers may require treatment with anti-tuberculosis medications.

Does the pt have gross hematuria?
60% of these pts present with microscopic hematuria, or gross hematuria.

What is this pt's occupation?
Occupational exposure to asbestos, cadmium, and solvents can be associated with renal cell carcinoma (RCC).

Does the pt smoke?
A twofold increase in risk for RCC exists in cigarette smokers in comparison with nonsmokers. The mechanism for this association is unclear.

Does any person in the pt's family have Von Hippel-Lindau disease (VHL)?
VHL is strongly associated with RCC, which develops in about 33% of pts with VHL disease.

Does the pt have renal failure?
The risk of pts who are on hemodialysis to acquire RCC is 8%, which is 50-fold higher than the general population.

Does the pt have gross hematuria and/or flank pain?
The classic triad for renal cell carcinoma is gross hematuria, flank pain, and a palpable abdominal mass.

Perform a physical examination
Physical exam can be benign in these pts, except for the presence of microscopic hematuria. The pt may be pale secondary to anemia (normochromic).

Palpate abdomen for masses
A palpable abdominal mass may be found (15% of pts).

Evaluate for cough and shortness of breath
Cough and shortness of breath may be secondary to lung metastasis.

Perform imaging studies
Intravenous pyelogram (IVP)
  • Can be ordered in the initial evaluation of pts with microscopic hematuria. Any suspicious masses should be confirmed with CT scan.

CT scan
  • Masses suspicious for RCC will enhance on CT when IV contrast is given. This is the test of choice for staging renal cell carcinoma because of the superior visualization of renal anatomy.

MRI
  • Superior to CT scan if vascular involvement (inferior vena cava) is suspected.

Perform diagnostic cystoscopy
Can help to differentiate the site of hematuria. Blood coming from the ureteral orifices is indicative of pathologic conditions above the bladder.

Perform urinalysis
Will reveal hematuria in 40% of cases.

Obtain bone scan if serum alkaline phosphatase level is elevated
Bone scan is obtained in pts with elevated alkaline phosphatase to rule out bone metastasis. Positive findings are confirmed with x-rays of the specific location.

Obtain laboratory studies
CBC: evaluate for anemia (normochromic).
Serum chemistries: evaluate renal and hepatic function.
Erythrocyte sedimentation rate: elevated in 70% of pts with RCC.

Microhematuria from RCC

Consider paraneoplastic syndrome

Pts with anemia, erythrocytosis, hypercalcemia, hypertension, and hepatic dysfunction should be evaluated for paraneoplastic syndromes secondary to RCC.

Definition of paraneoplastic syndrome

The presentation can be confusing, especially for those pts who present with paraneoplastic syndrome.

- Hypertension is seen in 40% and is refractory to antihypertensive therapy.
- Hypercalcemia occurs in 20% of pts, and is related to a parathyroid hormone related peptide.
- Erythrocytosis and hepatic dysfunction are also seen in this syndrome.

Consider an inherited form of RCC

RCC is either inherited or sporadic. Pts with inherited RCC may have associated diseases, such as VHL or hereditary papillary renal carcinoma.

Surgical excision

Surgical excision is the only curative treatment for RCC.

- Radical nephrectomy or partial nephrectomy can be considered the treatments of choice.

    - Partial nephrectomy is appropriate for pts with small (<4 cm) tumors, especially in the lower pole as well as bilateral tumors and tumors in pts with impaired renal function.

Consider chemotherapy regimens for metastatic RCC

Various hormonal and cytotoxic chemotherapeutic agents have been tried with little success.

- Immunotherapy with biologic response modifiers such as interleukin-2 and interferon-alpha are currently being studied.

S **Does the pt report any symptoms that could be associated with the mass?**
Perform a careful review of systems with pt to identify any possible symptoms that
could be linked to the incidental finding.
  • Possible symptoms include:
    ◆ Headaches
    ◆ Flushing

Review imagines study obtained (because this is an incidental finding)
CT scan: can assess whether masses are cystic or solid.

  • Benign adrenal cysts have thin, nonenhancing walls with fluid attenuation.
  • Malignant adrenal lesions are large, hemorrhagic or necrotic.
  • Masses with gross fat on CT (HU <30) are benign nonfunctional lesions.

MRI: can identify benign and malignant adrenal masses.

  • Chemical shift imaging can identify adrenal adenoma.
  • T2-weighted image that shows a high-intensity signal suggests pheochromocy-
    toma (light-bulb sign).

O **Perform a physical exam**
Observe general appearance.
  • Is the pt obese?
  • Do they appear as their stated age?
  • Is the appearance typical for their assigned gender?
    ◆ Increased facial hair in a female may suggest hormonal abnormalities as seen
      with adrenal masses (virilization).

Consider additional studies
24-hour urine catecholamine levels for metanephrine, vanillylmandelic acid, and
homovanillylmandelic acid to rule out pheochromocytoma.
Percutaneous CT-guided biopsy may be appropriate:
  • Pts with imaging characteristics suspicious for a metastatic lesion (example:
    woman with breast cancer who has an incidental adrenal mass on follow-up
    imaging study)
Exploratory surgery is suggested in pts with lesions > 5 cm on CT or MRI because
these techniques tend to underestimate adrenal lesions.

Incidental Adrenal Mass

Definition

Adrenal incidentalomas are silent adrenal masses found on CT or MRI scanning by chance. These masses are found in 0.6% to 4% of pts who have an abdominal CT. These masses may be cystic or solid, and are nonfunctional.

Differential diagnosis

- Adenoma
- Lymphoma
- Neuroblastoma
- Hematoma
- Adrenal hyperplasia
- Granulomatous disease
- Metastasis
- Pheochromocytoma
- Adrenal cortical carcinoma
- Adrenal myelolipoma
- Adrenal cyst
- Hemangioma

Determine functionality of the lesion.

Adrenal carcinomas are classified as:

- **Functional:** those tumors that produce hormones: Cushing's syndrome, hyperaldosteronism, feminizing syndromes in men, and virilization in females—increased testosterone, and increased DHEA 17-ketosteroids.
    - A limited evaluation is done for these pts, which includes potassium levels for hypertensive pts.
    - Glucocorticoid levels for pts with Cushing's syndrome and virilization.
    - 24-hour urine for catecholamines to rule out pheochromocytoma.
- **Nonfunctional:** those tumors that are hormonally inactive: incidentalomas.

Consider treatment options based on size of lesion

Greater than 6 cm and solid:

- Adrenalectomy

Greater than 6 cm and cystic:

- Consider CT-guided aspiration of cyst, and follow every 6 months. If repeat CT suggests cyst remains stable, continue to follow. If cyst enlarges, limited evaluation for functional masses, and remove cyst.
- Follow-up evaluation every 6 months. Continue to follow if cyst remains stable. Repeat limited evaluation for functional masses, and remove if cyst enlarges.

Less than 6 cm and solid: MRI

- High signal on T2-weighted image: adrenalectomy.
- Low signal on T2-weighted image: follow every 6 months as above.

Less than 6 cm and cystic:

- Follow every 6 months as above.

Does the pt complain of headaches, chest pain, and sweating?
The classic triad of symptoms for pheochromocytoma is headache, sweating, and palpitations.

Does the pt have a history of hypertension?
Hypertension is the most consistent sign and is secondary to catecholamine release (norepinephrine and epinephrine).
- 10% of pts with a pheochromocytoma may be normotensive.

Does the pt have any constitutional signs?
Additional signs and symptoms include pallor, flushing, tachycardia, chest pain, abdominal pain, and postural hypotension.

Is there a family history of pheochromocytoma or endocrine disease?
90% to 95% of pheochromocytoma is sporadic; however, in 5% to 10% of cases, it can be familial (multiple endocrine neoplasia [MEN] syndrome).

Perform a physical exam

General

Observe pt for signs of anxiety during encounter.
Increased catecholamines stimulate anxious behavior.

Check vital signs (including blood pressure and pulse)
Pheochromocytoma can be associated with systolic and diastolic hypertension.
Postural hypotension can also occur.
Look for signs of flushing.
Tachycardia is common.

Obtain pt's weight
Weight loss is associated with neoplastic conditions. Consider adrenocortical tumors or metastasis.

Carefully assess skin condition
Assess for dermatologic conditions: café-au-lait macules, neurofibromas, port wine stains, facial angiofibromas, ash-leaf hypopigmented macules, and small hypopigmented area (confetti sign).

Obtain 24-hour urine studies
24-hour urine for catecholamines (vanillylmandelic acid and homovanillylmandelic acid) and urinary levels of metanephrine.

Perform urinalysis
A urinalysis may reveal hematuria in 50% of cases, especially with pheochromocytoma of the urinary bladder.

Perform MRI
MRI: should be the initial scanning procedure.
- Provides good anatomic information.
- Images in both coronal and sagittal planes.
- May see increased enhancement of the lesion (light bulb sign) on T2-weighted study.

Consider CT scan
CT has >90% accuracy for detection of suprarenal masses, but cannot differentiate between pheochromocytoma and other adrenal masses.

Consider meta-iodobenzylguanidine (MIBG) scan
MIBG scintigraphy: good technique for finding residual or multiple pheochromocytomas because it seems to be more sensitive than CT for extra-adrenal masses.

Pheochromocytoma

Definition

Pheochromocytomas are typically benign adrenal mass lesions or masses that secrete catecholamines and cause symptoms of hypertension, anxiety, flushing, headaches, and palpitations.

Differential diagnosis

Symptoms can mimic eclampsia, toxemia of pregnancy, thyrotoxicosis, and generalized anxiety disorder.

Also consider: lymphoma, neuroblastoma, adrenal hyperplasia, granulomatous disease (tuberculosis), and simple adrenal cysts.

Remember the rule of tens for pheochromocytoma
10% extra-adrenal, 10% malignant, 10% in children, 10% familial, 10% bilateral

 Begin preoperative evaluation

All pts with pheochromocytoma should have a complete cardiac evaluation with echocardiogram and radionuclide scans before surgery, and should be screened for MEN syndromes.

Consider presurgical treatment with an alpha blocker

Pre-surgical treatment requires at least 4 weeks of alpha-adrenergic blockade (phenoxybenzamine) to obtain good blood pressure control.

- Beta-blockers (propranolol) are used in combination with alpha-adrenergic blockers in pts with arrhythmias.
- Alpha-methylparatyrosine is also recommended preoperatively with phenoxybenzamine and propranolol to decrease catecholamine production.

Surgery

Surgical removal of the tumor is the definitive treatment, except in pregnant pts. Tumors < 5 cm can be removed laparoscopically. Tumors > 5 cm may require an open surgical procedure.

Overall prognosis

Good. Surgical deaths are rare. BP returns to normal after surgery. Pts with persistent hypertension need further evaluation.

Does the pt have hematuria?
80% of pts present with gross, painless hematuria.
- 20% of pts present with microhematuria.

Does the pt have back or flank pain?
Pts with metastatic disease usually present with back or flank pain from metastasis to bone, retroperitoneum, or from ureteral obstruction.

Does the pt have symptoms of a urinary tract infection?
Approximately 30% of pts present with dysuria and irritative voiding symptoms.
- Urinalysis may reveal a urinary tract infection in 30% of pts.

Has the pt undergone any recent imaging studies?
Bladder cancer can metastasize to bone, liver, lymph nodes, and lungs.
- These pts should have a CT scan of the abdomen and pelvis, chest x-ray, and bone scan.

Were any recent laboratory studies performed?
Elevated liver function test results can indicate metastasis to the liver and or bone. Elevated creatinine may suggest ureteral obstruction from tumor.

Perform a physical examination

Evaluate for supraclavicular adenopathy
Those who have physical symptoms may present with:

| - palpable suprapubic abdominal mass | - hepatomegaly |
| - supraclavicular lymphadenopathy | - lymphedema |

Perform urinalysis
Should be performed in any pt complaining of voiding symptoms or gross hematuria.
- A urine cytologic exam should be included for pts with hematuria to evaluate the presence of malignant cells.

Perform diagnostic cystoscopy with biopsies
This procedure can be used for diagnosis and staging of bladder cancer.

Perform intravenous pyelography
Intravenous pyelography (IVP) can detect a filling defect in the bladder 60% of the time.
- Small tumors rarely detected by IVP.
- Ideally should be obtained prior to transurethral resection.

Perform CT with contrast
Very useful in clinical staging of pts with advanced bladder carcinoma.
- May demonstrate thickening of the bladder wall, extravesical extension, nodal involvement, or distant metastasis.

Consider metastatic workup
Consists of chest x-ray and bone scan.
- Chest x-ray is the initial screening for pulmonary metastasis.
- Bone scan is obtained in pts with invasive or locally advanced tumors and skeletal symptoms or elevated serum alkaline phosphatase.

A   **Metastatic Bladder Carcinoma**

Muscle invasive bladder carcinomas are considered at much higher risk for metastatic disease.

- These pts may be N+, as well as M+ for staging.
- Metastatic bladder carcinoma has 50% mortality rate, even with treatment.
- Obturator and external iliac lymph nodes commonly involved.

23% to 43% of pts achieve a complete response to chemotherapy alone.

P   **Treatment**

Consider surgical therapy

Transurethral resection of bladder tumor (TURBT) alone.

- May be curative in select pts with low-grade, localized invasive disease.
- Recurrences develop in 50% of pts.
- Repeat TURBT with biopsy recommended to determine presence of redidual disease.

External beam radiotherapy.

- Favored in Europe as curative therapy.
- 20% may require salvage cystectomy.
- 5-year survival rate is 30%.

Radical cystectomy.

- Radical cystectomy and urinary diversion.
- Urethrectomy added if tumor involves prostatic urethra in males and bladder neck in females.
- Various types of diversion procedures (continent vs. incontinent).

Consider adjuvant chemotherapy and/or radiotherapy.

- Invasion of adjacent tissue (T4, N+, or M+). These pts are treated with systemic chemotherapy followed by either surgery or radiation therapy.
- Recommended chemotherapy is the MVAC protocol—methotrexate, doxorubicin (Adriamycin), and cisplatin.

S

What is the age and racial background of the pt?
The most common occurrence of penile cancer is people in their 60s.

- A much higher prevalence in the African and South American population (20% of malignant lesions tend to be penile carcinoma).
- Penile carcinoma rarely presents in children.

Has the pt been circumcised? What are his hygiene practices?

Improper/poor hygiene is the number one etiologic factor associated with penile cancer.

- Penile smegma in the uncircumcised male can accumulate and build up under the foreskin, causing chronic irritation, which can potentially lead to carcinotic formation.

Is the pt sexually active/any STD history?
Human papilloma virus (HPV) has been noted in correlation with penile carcinoma.

- Reports of subclinical HPV infections are common, especially in male sexual partners of females with a history of in situ or cervical carcinoma.

O

Perform a physical examination

Examine the shaft and glans penis
Bowen's disease and erythroplasia of Queyrat present as erythema of the glans and shaft, respectively.

Are penile ulcerations present?
Squamous cell carcinoma is most common type (98% of all cases), and comprises the majority of penile cancers.

- Usually originates on the glans, then prepuce and shaft.
- May present as papillary or ulcerative in appearance.

Is there evidence of induration, erythema, or nodules?
Small areas of induration/erythema, ulceration, small nodule, exophytic growth on the penis.

Order laboratory tests
Lab evaluation is typically normal, with a potential for anemia and leukocytosis secondary to chronic disease or spreading local infection.

- Hypercalcemia is seen in 20% of pts with no osseous metastases, and can be correlated with the volume of disease.

Perform radiologic evaluation for metastasis
A proper metastatic workup should include CXR, bone scan, and CT scan of abdomen and pelvis.

- All performed to assess staging and spread of the cancer.

Penile Carcinoma

Consider the differential diagnosis

Chancre secondary to syphilis infection commonly presents as non-painful ulcerations on the glans and shaft.

- Chancroid presents as a painful ulceration, and pt needs to be tested for *Haemophilus.*
- Condylomata acuminata appear as "grape cluster" lesions, which can be identified via biopsy.

Stage the cancer after results of biopsy and surgical resection

Stage I: Tumor is confined to the glans or prepuce

Stage II: Tumor involves the penile shaft

Stage III: Operable inguinal node metastasis

Stage IV: Tumor extends beyond the shaft, with inoperable inguinal or distant metastases

Consider circumcision for lesions of the prepuce

If the pt is uncircumcised, and the lesion is on contained on the prepuce, a circumcision may be sufficient.

Consider topical therapy for superficial lesions

Topical 5-fluorouracil cream may be appropriate.

Consider radiotherapy for superficial lesions

Radiation is also a possible treatment for superficial lesions, which will preserve erectile function, with a high cure rate.

- Potential candidates for radiation: small (<3 cm), superficial, exophytic lesions or noninvasive cancers on the glans or coronal sulcus
- Pts are at increased risk of developing fistulas, and urethral stenosis.

Consider partial penectomy or total penectomy

If the lesion is on the glans or shaft and is invasive, the area must be excised via partial or complete penectomy which is the standard of care.

- A 2-cm margin is necessary for a complete removal of the cancer. Otherwise, there is increased risk of recurrence.

Consider antibiotic therapy initially for inguinal adenopathy

Enlargement of lymph nodes does not necessarily equate with metastasis. In 50% of cases, enlargement is due to inflammation and not carcinoma invasion.

- The primary lesion should be treated, and a 4 to 6 week course of antibiotics for inguinal lymphatics.
- If the inflammation persists, ilioinguinal lymph node dissection should be performed.

Treat pts with disseminated disease with chemotherapy

Pts with disseminated disease are treated with chemotherapy: bleomycin, methotrexate, cisplatin, and 5-fluorouracil.

S **What is the age, ethnicity, and gender of the pt?**

The occurrence of urethral cancer is most prevalent in white females in the seventh decade of life.

- African Americans, although less likely to develop this malignancy, have a markedly worse prognosis.

Does the pt have any history of bladder cancer or STD/HPV history?
One of the few correlations that have been linked to urethral cancer with previous bladder cancer and prior STD history, especially HPV exposure.

Does the pt have hematuria, dyspareunia, discharge, hematospermia (men), or swelling?
These symptoms have all been associated with urethral carcinoma.

Are there any irritative or obstructive voiding symptoms?

These symptoms are usually associated with benign stricture, but may also be evidence of a urethral neoplasm.

Any complaints of urinary incontinence?
Can be caused by bladder outlet obstruction secondary to tumor blockage, which can lead to overflow incontinence, and the constant feeling of a full bladder.

O **Perform a physical examination**

Carefully examine the genitalia for nodules
Firm nodule(s) along the perineum, labia, or glans/shaft of the penis may be identified.

Is there any evidence of abscess formation?
Evaluate for signs of tissue necrosis/urethral abscess.

Is there a fistula?
Fistula formation (urethral-cutaneous or urethral-vaginal) is possible.

Is there a palpable urethral mass?
Urethral diverticula can be associated with urethral carcinoma.

Evaluate for genital ulcers
Penile or vaginal ulcers can be found.

Evaluate for lymphadenopathy
Palpable lymph nodes may represent metastases or inflammation.

Perform laboratory studies
- Urinalysis/urine cytology   - CBC
- Alkaline phosphatase   - Serum electrolytes

Perform imaging studies
CXR
CT abdomen, pelvis, perineum/MRI (not cost effective, but increasingly popular)

A **Urethral carcinoma**

Determine cancer type

In men and women, squamous cell cancer is most common, followed by transitional cell carcinoma.

- In men, the most common sites are membranobulbar and penile regions of the urethra. Transitional cell carcinoma occurs in the prostatic urethra.

P **Perform cystoscopy and biopsy**

Perform cystoscopy and biopsy to determine histology and staging.

Surgical resection

Primary method of treatment of urethral cancer.

The extent of invasive surgery is based upon the tumor location, as well as the classification and staging.

Consider local excision

For localized, low-grade, distal urethral neoplasms in men.

Consider partial penectomy

Partial penectomy for infiltrative, distally occurring lesions urethra.

Consider radical (total) penectomy

Radical (total) penectomy: if proximal 1/2 urethra is positive for infiltrating tumor.
Pelvic lymphadenectomy with en bloc pts with T2/Nx/M0 or higher tumors in the bulbomembranous or prostatic urethra.

Consider pelvic exenteration in women

Because of the short urethra in women, consider pelvic exenteration procedure (radical cystectomy, urethrectomy and urinary diversion).

Consider radiation therapy

Superficial tumors can be treated with radiation alone, or with surgical removal of the neoplastic lesion.

- Often used in pts who refuse surgical therapy.

Consider chemotherapy

Multiagent chemotherapy with methotrexate, vinblastine, doxorubicin, and cisplatin has been used in various combinations, and studies have shown that a combined therapeutic had the best results.

What is the age, ethnicity, and gender of the pt?

The male-female ratio is 2.7:1, respectively, with the disease being more common in Caucasians than in African Americans.

- The peak incidence of diagnosis at 65 years old and incidence increases steadily with age.
- Women and African Americans have a worse prognosis when diagnosed with bladder carcinoma.

Does the pt smoke? Did the pt smoke in the past?

50% of males and 31% of females diagnosed with bladder cancer were smokers.

What is the pt's employment history?

People employed in, or that have chronic contact with chemical, dye, rubber, petroleum, leather, and printing services have an increased incidence of bladder cancer.

Is there a history of gross or microscopic hematuria?

All cases of hematuria are assumed to be bladder cancer unless proven otherwise. All pts with hematuria need evaluation of their upper and lower urinary tracts.

Perform a physical examination

Physical exam may be normal.

Those pts who have symptoms may present with a palpable suprapubic mass, or a rectal mass on digital rectal examination (DRE) from tumor extension to rectum.

- Hepatomegaly, supraclavicular lymphadenopathy, and lymphedema may be identified.

Perform urinalysis

Should be performed in any pt complaining of voiding symptoms or gross hematuria.

Perform urine cytology

Cells for microscopic examination are collected from voided urine.

- Urine cytology is 30% sensitive in diagnosing low-grade bladder cancer but is excellent for detecting carcinoma in situ (CIS) and high-grade lesions (90%).

Obtain images study of the upper tract

Hematuria can result from upper urinary tract sources.

- Must evaluate the kidneys and ureters.
- Consider intravenous pyelography.
- CT scan is an acceptable upper urinary tract imaging study.

Transitional Cell Carcinoma (TCC)
TCC is the most prevalent bladder cancer (90%).
- Usually found as papillary, exophytic lesions, which tend to be superficial.
- 50%–70% of bladder tumors are superficial (maximal invasion into lamina propria).

Differential diagnosis
Transitional cell carcinoma (90%)
Squamous cell carcinoma (7%–8%)
Adenocarcinoma (1–2%)
Other types: (<1%)
- Small cell carcinoma
- Sarcoma
- Melanoma
- Carcinoid tumor

Stage the tumor after cystoscopy and bladder biopsy:
Ta: papillary tumor that is restricted to the epithelium
T1: invasion is limited to the lamina propria
T2: invasion into the bladder muscle
- Clinical staging has a strong tendency to underestimate the metastatic spread in approximately 53% of pts.

 Cystoscopy, bladder biopsy and transurethral resection of bladder tumor
Allows for diagnosis and treatment of this superficial lesion.

Consider intravesical chemotherapy
Appropriate for multifocal superficial and recurrent disease.
Also appropriate for carcinoma in situ and high-grade TCC initially involving the lamina propria.

Choose the appropriate intravesical agent for chemotherapy
Mitomycin C: inhibits DNA synthesis.
Thiotepa: serves as an alkylating agent.
Bacillus Calmette-Guérin immunotherapy is the preferred therapy in treating superficial bladder cancer.
- A live attenuated form of *Mycobacterium bovis* is introduced into the bladder.
- Mucosal ulceration and granuloma formation are typical.
- Induction therapy is given once per week for 6 weeks.

Set surveillance protocol
Pts will be followed with periodic cystoscopic evaluations, urine cytology, and upper tract imaging studies.

II

Sexual and Voiding Dysfunction

S   **When does the pt leak urine?**

Stress urinary incontinence (SUI) is associated with leakage of urine during increases in intra-abdominal pressure (i.e., coughing, sneezing, or Valsalva maneuver).

Does the pt leak urine on any other occasion?
Up to 50% of women with SUI may have a component of urge incontinence.
A pt with urge incontinence will leak urine when they have a strong desire to void but cannot make it to the rest room in time.

What is the primary component to the pt's incontinence?
If women complain more about leaking urine when they cough, sneeze or stand up, treating their stress incontinence might cure their urge component as well.
   • If urge incontinence is their primary component, then you will need to focus on treating their urge incontinence and stress incontinence as separate entities.

How many pads does the pt use a day?
Quantifying the number of pads used will help the physician determine the severity of SUI.

Does the pt have any other urinary symptoms or signs such as urgency or frequency?
Assess for irritative symptoms such as frequency, urgency, dysuria, and nocturia.
   • Assess for gross hematuria.

   • Pts with SUI may have urge and/or urge incontinence.
   • These pts generally do not have any irritative urinary symptoms.

Has the pt had vaginal surgeries or vaginal deliveries?
Conditions associated with SUI include multiple vaginal deliveries, obesity, previous pelvic surgery, or pelvic radiation.

O   **Perform a physical exam**

Perform provocative testing to demonstrate urine leakage
Assess for leakage of urine when the pt coughs or performs a Valsalva maneuver. Make sure the pt has a full bladder.
   • If the pt voids before this test, she may not demonstrate SUI because the bladder will be empty.

Assess urethral hypermobility
Assess for hypermobility of the urethra and bladder when the pt coughs or performs a Valsalva maneuver.
   • Determine if the pt has a cystocele or rectocele

Consider urodynamics
Urodynamic evaluation can be performed. The Valsalva leak point pressure (VLPP) determines the amount of abdominal pressure that leads to leakage of urine.
   • The lower the VLPP, the more severe the SUI.

Stress Urinary Incontinence
Stress incontinence is the leakage of urine that occurs with increases in abdominal pressure.

Classify and grade SUI (based on video urodynamic studies)
Grade 0
- Closed bladder neck and proximal urethra at rest. With increased intra-abdominal pressure, the bladder neck and proximal urethra open. The pt does not leak urine.

Grade I
- Closed bladder neck that is located above the inferior margin of the pubic symphysis at rest. With stress, the bladder neck and proximal urethra open and descend less than 2 cm. The pt leaks urine.

Grade IIa
- Closed bladder neck that is located above the inferior margin of the pubic symphysis at rest. With stress, the bladder neck opens and descends greater than 2 cm. The pt leaks urine.

Grade IIb
- Closed bladder neck that is located at or below the inferior margin of the pubic symphysis at rest. With stress, the bladder neck opens and the pt leaks urine. The bladder neck may or may not descend with stress.

Grade III
- Intrinsic sphincter deficiency: The bladder neck and proximal urethra are open at rest.

P **Assess degree of pt's bother by their symptoms**
Pts with mild leakage of urine and low degree of bother from their symptoms are best managed with pelvic floor exercises (Kegel exercises).

Consider medical treatment
Medical treatment options include imipramine and phenylephrine. These drugs work by increasing bladder outlet resistance.
- These drugs have limited success in the management of SUI.

Consider vaginal estrogen creams
Estrogen creams can increase mucosal coaptation of the urethra and increase bladder outlet resistance in pts with atrophic vaginitis and stress incontinence.

Consider surgical treatment
Surgical treatment options have the highest success rate in SUI. Surgical options include injection of periurethral bulking agents, bladder suspension procedures and sling procedures.
- Sling procedures are the standard of care for SUI.
- Assocciated prolapse (cystocele or rectocele) can also be repaired.

S   **When does the pt leak urine?**

The pt with postprostatectomy incontinence will have leakage of urine during increases in intra-abdominal pressure.

Does the pt leak urine on any other occasion?
A pt with postprostatectomy incontinence will have stress incontinence as the etiology.
- A postprostatectomy pt may get a bladder neck contracture or an anastomotic stricture, which can lead to urge or overflow incontinence.
- Rarely, a pt can form a fistula after a pelvic surgery, such as a radical retropubic prostatectomy, leading to total incontinence.

Was the pt continent before his prostatectomy?
If a pt was incontinent before the surgery, he will be incontinent after the surgery. This type of pt may have urge or overflow incontinence in addition to his stress urinary incontinence.

How many pads does the pt use per day?
Quantifying the number of pads used per day will help determine the severity of pt's incontinence.

Has the pt's incontinence been getting better, worse, or the same as time has progressed from their surgery?

Most pts with postprostatectomy incontinence will show some improvement in their symptoms within the first year after their prostatectomy.

O   **Perform a physical exam**

Incite urine leakage with provocative maneuvers
Assess for leakage of urine when the pt coughs or performs a Valsalva maneuver. Make sure the pt has a full bladder.

Obtain postvoid residual
Can help rule out bladder outlet obstruction or inadequate bladder contraction.

Consider uroflow evaluation
Can help assess for bladder outlet resistance.

Consider urodynamic evaluation
Urodynamics can be performed.
The Valsalva leak point pressure (VLPP) tells you the amount of abdominal pressure that leads to leakage of urine. The lower the pt's VLPP, the more severe his stress incontinence.

Postprostatectomy incontinence

Sphincteric dysfunction

Sphincteric dysfunction accounts for the majority of the postprostatectomy pt's incontinence.

During a radical prostatectomy, the proximal (internal) urethral sphincter is removed. These pts rely solely on the distal urethral sphincter to maintain continence.

- These pts generally have stress urinary incontinence, but they can have urge or overflow incontinence if there is bladder outlet obstruction from an anastomotic stricture or a bladder neck contracture.

Bladder instability

Occasionally after radical prostatectomy, pts will complain of urge incontinence with high pressure voiding. This can be a result of surgery.

Diagnosis can be made with urodynamics.

Treat the pt according to symptoms and degree of bother

For stress incontinence after a prostatectomy, the pt should perform pelvic floor exercises on a regular basis.

- The mean time for a return to continence after a radical prostatectomy is 16 weeks but most physicians will give a pt up to 1 year to achieve continence before offering additional treatment options.

Consider medical therapy

Medical therapy has little success in men with sudden urge incontinence after prostatectomy.

- Imipramine improves incontinence in approximately 35% of pts.
- Duloxetine is an agent in phase III trials that may show promise in treatment of male postprostatectomy incontinence.

Consider surgical treatments

Surgical treatments are the most effective for stress incontinence after a prostatectomy.

- Surgical options include injection of periurethral bulking agents (collagen), artificial urinary sphincters and sling procedures.
  - Artificial urinary sphincter involves placement of a synthetic cuff around the bladder neck/proximal urethra; the cuff remains inflated until intentional deflation by a scrotal or labial pump.
  - Success rate of 80% to 90%.
  - Complications include erosion, device failure, and intraoperative injury to the urethra, infection, and device failure.
- Urge or overflow incontinence can be treated by incising or dilating any anastomotic strictures or bladder neck contractures that are causing bladder outlet obstruction.

S   **When does the pt leak urine?**

Urge incontinence occurs when a pt gets an intense urge to urinate and cannot hold their urine long enough to get to a restroom.

Does the pt leak urine on other occasions?
Pts can also have stress urinary incontinence along with their urge incontinence.

How many pads does the pt use a day?
Quantifying the number of pads used will help the physician determine the severity of her incontinence.

Does the pt have any other urinary symptoms?
Assess for irritative symptoms such as frequency, urgency, dysuria, and nocturia. Assess for gross hematuria.
  • Irritative voiding symptoms also occur in pts with transitional cell carcinoma of the bladder.

Does the pt have any neurologic conditions associated with urgency or urge incontinence?
Upper motor neuron lesions are associated with detrusor hyperreflexia.

   Perform a physical exam

Perform provocative testing to determine sudden urge incontinence (SUI)
Assess for leakage of urine with cough or Valsalva maneuver. Up to 50% of pts with SUI will have urgency as well.

Perform a careful neurologic examination
Do a neurologic exam especially focusing on anal sphincter tone, bulbocavernous reflex, deep tendon reflexes, and strength and sensation in the extremities.

Perform urodynamic testing
Urodynamics can be performed. The detrusor leak point pressure (DLPP) will determine you how much pressure generated from an involuntary detrusor contraction causes the pt to leak urine.

A   **Urge urinary incontinence**

Definition

Urge incontinence refers to the leakage of urine with involuntary contractions of the bladder.

- The lower the DLPP, the more severe the urge incontinence.

Differential diagnosis

Idiopathic
Cerebrovascular accident
Parkinson's disease
Spinal cord injury
Multiple sclerosis
Brain tumor
Dementia

P   **Treatment options**

Consider medical therapies

Anticholinergic medications are the mainstay of treatment in urge incontinence.

- Oxybutynin chloride (Ditropan)
  - Antimuscarinic and anticholinergic agent
  - Significant improvement in urinary frequency, urge incontinence episodes and pt satisfaction when compared to placebo.
  - Caution of use in pts with angle closure glaucoma.
  - Immediate release and extended release forms
- Tolterodine tartrate (Detrol)
  - Antimuscarinic agent with detrusor selectivity over salivary glands
  - Significant improvement in urinary frequency, urge incontinence episodes, and pt satisfaction when compared to placebo
  - Caution of use in pts with angle closure glaucoma.
  - Immediate release and extended release forms
- Oxybutynin transdermal (Oxytrol)
  - Antimuscarinic and anticholinergic agent
  - Significant improvement in urinary frequency, urgency incontinence, and pt satisfaction
  - Less anticholinergic side effects than oral agents
  - Patch application changed twice weekly but associated with erythema and itchiness at patch side in 15% of pts.

Recently approved agents solafenacin (Vesicare), darifenacin (Enablex), trospium chloride (Sanctura) are effective in treatment of urge incontinence.

Consider behavioral therapies

Behavioral therapy with timed voids and a voiding diary can lead to successful management of urge incontinence.

Consider sacral neuromodulation

Sacral neuromodulation (Interstim) is considered a second-line therapy for pts with refractory urge incontinence and urgency/frequency.

- Bladder pacemaker with electrode placed into S3 foramina
- Test implant placed followed by permanent implant if positive response obtained.
- Results include 50% reduction in urge incontinence episodes, 50% reduction in urinary frequency, 50% improvement in voided volume as well as improved quality of life data.

S What is the pt's chief complaint?

Pts with Peyronie's disease usually complain of curvature of the penis.

Does the pt experience pain with erections?

Two-thirds of pts with Peyronie's disease will experience pain with erection.

Which direction does the penis curve and where on the penis does the curve begin?

This helps let the physician know where on the penis the pathology lies. Dorsal and ventral curvatures are approached differently from an operative prospective.

When did the pt first notice this condition?

This lets the physician know if the onset was sudden or insidious.

Does the curvature prevent sexual activity?

Pts with severe curvature might not be able to penetrate the vagina due to the severe angulation of their penis.

Does the pt have any problems obtaining or maintaining erections?

Pts with Peyronie's disease may have a component of erectile dysfunction because the plaque on the tunica albuginea might not provide adequate compression of emissary veins resulting in venous leakage of blood from the corpora cavernosa.

- Leakage of blood from the corpora will result in a less rigid erection and/or possibly no erection at all.

Does the pt have any history of penile trauma?

Trauma to the penis can lead to plaque formation in the tunica albuginea.
- Plaque formation leads to decreased elasticity of the tunica and curvature of the penis.

Has the pt ever been treated for this condition in the past?

It is important to know what treatment options the pt has already tried to determine a treatment plan for the pt at this time.
- Conservative treatments that failed in the past are likely to fail again.

O Perform a physical exam

Examine the penis for plaque formation

Most plaques are located on the dorsal surface of the penis.

Assess degree of curvature

Assess for curvature of the penis even though most pts with Peyronie's have curvature only when the penis is in the erect state.

Assess chordee

Assess for chordee because this can lead to ventral curvature of the penis.

Assess for Dupuytren's contracture

Dupuytren's contractures are associated with Peyronie's disease.

A **Peyronie's disease**
Peyronie's disease is the formation of a calcified plaque in the tunica albuginea leading to curvature of the penis.
- Some pts may have pain with erection as well.
- Plaque forms secondary to trauma to penis. In most cases, the inciting trauma is related to sexual activity.

P **Treatment options**

Consider medical management
Medical management with oral colchicine, vitamin E, para-aminobenzoic acid (PABA), or intralesional verapamil can be performed.
- Success rates for these procedures is approximately 50% to 60%
- Some treatments require the pts to take large numbers of pills each day. For example, pts treated with PABA will ingest 32 pills/day.
- Intralesional verapamil injections require pts to undertake a series of 8 to 12 biweekly injections.

Consider treatment for erectile dysfunction
Many pts with Peyronie's disease have erectile dysfunction (ED). For those pts with minimal to moderate curvature that does not prohibit penetration, treatment of ED with agents such as sildenafil, vardenafil, or tadalafil can be considered.

Consider surgical repair
Surgical repair is indicated for severe curvature.
- Some pts have an underlying ED that is refractory to conventional therapy.
- Pts ultimately may benefit from implantation of a penile prosthesis.

Carefully explain the risks of surgical repair
Risks of these surgical procedures can be significant and include
- Return of the penile plaque and curvature
- Penile shortening
- Penile numbness
- ED

Does the pt complain of irritative or obstructive voiding symptoms?
Assess for symptoms such as urgency, frequency, incomplete bladder emptying, or nocturia.

Does the pt ever leak urine?
See if the pt is incontinent when he/she gets the urge to void and cannot make it to the rest room in time (urge incontinence) or if the pt leaks urine without sensing that the bladder is full (overflow incontinence).

Does the pt have any established neurologic problems?
Many neurologic conditions can be associated with voiding dysfunction.

- Examples include brain tumor, dementia, Parkinson's disease, multiple sclerosis, stroke, and spinal cord injuries.

Does the pt have any extremity weakness, numbness, or the presence of fecal incontinence?
Complaints of these symptoms could alert the physician to an underlying neurologic condition that can be the cause of the pt's voiding symptoms.

Perform a physical exam

Perform a neurologic examination
Assess motor and sensory components of the extremities, anal tone, and the bulbo-cavernous reflex.

Obtain post-void residual
This test will assess how well the pt empties their bladder.

Obtain urodynamic evaluation
Assess what happens to the bladder as the bladder is being filled and when the pt voids.

- Urge incontinence occurs if the pt leaks urine with an uninhibited bladder contraction during filling.
- If the pt does not demonstrate bladder contractions when trying to void this suggests an atonic or hypocontractile bladder.

Neurogenic voiding dysfunction

Consider the differential diagnosis

Neurogenic voiding dysfunction results from a neurologic condition that causes abnormal function of the bladder.

- Neurologic lesions can cause detrusor hyperreflexia, impaired sphincteric relaxation (sphincter dyssynergia), or a hypocontractile/atonic bladder.

Consider the location of the neurologic lesion

Lesions above the pontine micturition center result in detrusor hyperreflexia.
Lesions between the pontine micturition center and the sacral spinal cord lead to hyperreflexia and sphincter dyssynergia.
Lesions below the sacral cord result in an atonic bladder

P **Treatment options**

Consider anticholinergic medications

Pts with detrusor hyperreflexia can be managed with anticholinergic medications.

- Oxybutynin chloride (Ditropan)
  - Antimuscarinic and anticholinergic agent
  - Significant improvement in urinary frequency, urge incontinence episodes, and pt satisfaction when compared to placebo.
  - Caution of use in pts with angle closure glaucoma.
  - Immediate release and extended release forms
- Tolterodine tartrate (Detrol)
  - Antimuscarinic agent with detrusor selectivity over salivary glands
  - Significant improvement in urinary frequency, urge incontinence episodes, and pt satisfaction when compared to placebo.
  - Caution of use in pts with angle closure glaucoma.
  - Immediate release and extended release forms
- Oxybutynin transdermal (Oxytrol)
  - Antimuscarinic and anticholinergic agent
  - Significant improvement in urinary frequency, urgency incontinence, and pt satisfaction.
  - Fewer anticholinergic side effects than oral agents.
  - Patch application changed twice weekly but associated with erythema and itchiness at patch side in 15% of pts.

Recently approved agents solafenacin (Vesicare), darifenacin (Enablex), trospium chloride (Sanctura) are effective in treatment of urge incontinence.

Consider clean intermittent catheterization

Atonic bladder is managed with clean intermittent catheterization (CIC) or an indwelling catheter.

- The goal is to prevent urinary stasis which can lead to infection or formation of calculi.
- Catheterization also prevents the bladder from filling beyond its capacity leading to overflow incontinence.
- Detrusor sphincter dyssynergia can be treated with alpha blockers, which relax the muscles of the bladder neck and sphincter. CIC may also be required.

Consider sacral neuromodulation

Sacral neuromodulation (Interstim) is considered a second-line therapy for pts with nonobstructive urinary retention, refractory urge incontinence, and urgency/frequency.

- Bladder pacemaker with electrode placed into S3 foramina
- Test implant placed followed by permanent implant if positive response obtained.
- Results include 50% reduction in urge incontinence episodes, 50% reduction in urinary frequency, 50% improvement in voided volume as well as improved quality of life data. May decrease or eliminate the need for CIC.

S   **Does the pt have irritative or obstructive voiding symptoms?**
Pts usually complain of a decrease in the force of their stream, incomplete emptying of their bladder, straining to void, hesitancy, terminal dribbling, and nocturia.

When did the pt's symptoms begin and how have they changed over time?
Benign prostatic hyperplasia (BPH) is a slow, ongoing process that worsens over time. The main risk factor for BPH is prostatic exposure to testosterone. Ninety percent of men over the age of 80 will experience BPH symptoms.

Does the pt have a history of urinary retention, bladder calculi, post–obstructive renal insufficiency, recurrent urinary tract infection (UTI)?
These problems indicate a more severe degree of BPH and are indications for surgical treatment of their prostatic hypertrophy.

How did the pt score on the IPSS or American Urology Association (AUA) symptom score questionnaire?
These are questionnaires that have been used to quantify pt's symptoms. Scores of 1 to 7: mild symptoms, 8 to 19: moderate symptoms, 20 to 35: severe symptoms.

What is the pt's degree of bother from his symptoms?
Pts are offered treatment options for BPH depending on the severity of their symptoms and their degree of bother from their symptoms.

What is the pt's prostate-specific antigen (PSA)?
PSA can correlate with prostate size. Increasing PSA values correlate with a higher rate of BPH-related complications such as urinary retention, urosepsis, renal insufficiency, and the need for BPH-related surgery.

O   **Perform a physical exam**

Evaluate prostate for size and the presence of nodules
Assess the size of the prostate, presence of any nodules, induration, asymmetry, or any tenderness. Keep in mind that prostate size doesn't correlate with symptom score or severity.

- Pts with small prostate glands may have severe symptoms and pts with large prostate glands may be without any voiding symptoms.

Obtain postvoid residual and uroflowmetry
Postvoid residual will assess how well the pt is emptying his bladder.
Uroflowmetry will assess how forceful the pt's urinary flow is.

Benign Prostatic Hyperplasia

Definition

BPH is the hyperplasia of the epithelial cells of the prostate that occurs secondary to exposure to testosterone/dihydrotestosterone.

- The enlarged prostate can cause bladder outlet obstruction and impede urination.
- At first, the detrusor muscle will hypertrophy to overcome the bladder outlet obstruction.
- Later on in the disease process, the detrusor will decompensate and will no longer be able to overcome the increased bladder outlet resistance.

Treatment options

Consider treatment with an alpha blocker

Alpha blockers are the primary medical treatment for BPH. They work by relaxing the smooth muscle of the prostate and bladder neck to decrease bladder outlet resistance.

- Examples include: tamsulosin (Flomax), doxazosin (Cardura), terazosin (Hytrin), and alfuzosin (Uroxitral)
  - Agents will improve pt symptoms and urinary flow rate when compared to placebo.
  - Alfuzosin and tamsulosin do not need to be dose titrated.
  - Typical adverse effects include asthenia and postural hypotension.
  - Do not reduce incidence of urinary retention, need for BPH-related surgery and renal insufficiency.

Consider treatment with a 5-alpha reductase inhibitor

5-alpha reductase inhibitors work by inhibiting the conversion of testosterone to dihydrotestosterone.

- Examples include finasteride (Proscar) and dutasteride (Avodart)
- This class of drugs has been found to be beneficial in pts with PSA values >1.5 ng/dL and prostate size greater than 40 g.
- Will reduce incidence of urinary retention, need for BPH related surgery and risk of renal insufficiency.

Consider surgical treatments

There are numerous surgical options for BPH. Transurethral resection of the prostate is the gold standard against which all other surgical options are judged.

- Surgery removes the tissue obstructing the urethral lumen. Indications for surgery include renal insufficiency secondary to BPH, recurrent UTI, bladder calculi, urinary retention secondary to BPH.

Consider minimally invasive surgical treatments

Minimally invasive treatments such as transurethral microwave therapy, water-induced thermotherapy, holmium laser prostate resections, and green-light laser prostatectomy have recently been popularized in the treatment of BPH.

- Long-term follow-up of these procedures is still unavailable.
- Short-term data suggest an improvement in urinary flow rate and AUA symptom score.

S **When was the last time the pt was able to sustain an erection firm enough for penetration and stay firm until orgasm was achieved?**
This lets the physician know when the pt began to have erectile dysfunction (ED).

Does the pt achieve nocturnal erections?
If the pt can achieve erections while asleep or awakens with an erection, then the pt has psychogenic ED.

Has the pt experienced erections with a different sexual partner?
If a pt is able to achieve and sustain erections with a different partner, then the pt has psychogenic ED.

Can the pt get firm enough to penetrate into his partner? Can he maintain rigidity until he reaches orgasm?
This helps the physician quantify how bad the pt's ED is. A pt that cannot achieve rigidity for penetration has a more severe case of ED than a pt that can penetrate his partner but experiences detumescence during intercourse.

How does the pt feel about the fact that he cannot maintain an erection during sexual activity?
If the pt is not bothered by his ED, you do not need to treat him.

How is the pt's libido?
Low sexual desire may be indicative of low testosterone levels.
Decreased libido may be one of the signs of depression.

What other medical problems does the pt have?
Other medical illnesses may cause ED. Causes of ED can be broken into vascular, neurogenic, hormonal/endocrine, psychogenic, idiopathic, and a combination of any of these factors.

Does the pt have a new onset of depression or anxiety?
Depression and anxiety can contribute to ED.

Does the pt have any a history of penile trauma or curvature to the penis?
Trauma to the penis can cause the development of a plaque in the tunica albuginea (Peyronie's disease). The penile plaque can cause curvature of the penis and prevent compression of emissary veins during an erection, which impedes the sequestering of blood in the penis to maintain an erection.

O **Perform a physical examination**

Perform a genitourinary examination
Assess sensation of the genitalia during the examination.
Assess for penile numbness.
Perform a digital rectal examination and evaluate the testes for masses.

Perform a vascular examination
Feel peripheral pulses to evaluate for peripheral vascular disease. Do a thorough neurologic exam to evaluate for neuropathy.

Obtain SHIM score (sexual health inventory for men) questionnaire
Scores less than 21 of a possible 25 indicate ED.

Consider nocturnal penile tumescence (NPT) testing
Measure nocturnal penile tumescence with a RIGScan, stamp test, or sleep laboratory study.
If pts can achieve a nocturnal erection, they have psychogenic ED.

Psychogenic erectile dysfunction

ED is the inability to maintain a satisfactory erection until orgasm is achieved. Psychogenic causes include depression, anxiety, and inability to be aroused.

P Treatment options

Consider treatment of the underlying medical problem

Treatment may include behavioral modification, biofeedback, antidepressants, and/or anxiolytics.

Consider first-line oral therapies

Oral PDE5 inhibitors (sildenafil, vardenafil, or tadalafil) are the first-line therapy for ED in pts without hormonal abnormalities.

- PDE5 inhibitors work by inhibiting the breakdown of cyclic guanosine monophosphate (GMP).
- Cyclic GMP promotes cavernosal smooth muscle relaxation.
- If a pt is not achieving erections with an oral agent, make sure they were using the agent properly and that they have tried the maximum recommended dose.

Consider second-line therapies

Second-line therapy includes the use of a vacuum erection device, intraurethral alprostadil, or intracavernosal alprostadil.

Alprostadil is a prostaglandin E1 agonist that causes cavernosal smooth muscle relaxation.

If pts fail the second-line therapies or they are uncomfortable using the second-line therapies, penile prosthesis may be considered.

S **When was the last time the pt was able to sustain an erection firm enough for penetration and stay firm until orgasm was achieved?**
This lets the physician know when the pt began to have erectile dysfunction (ED).

Does the pt achieve nocturnal erections?
If the pt can achieve erections while asleep or awakens with an erection, then the pt has psychogenic ED.

Has the pt experienced erections with a different sexual partner?
If a pt is able to achieve and sustain erections with a different partner, then the pt has psychogenic ED.

Can the pt get firm enough to penetrate into his partner? Can he maintain rigidity until he reaches orgasm?
This helps the physician quantify how bad the pt's ED is.
- A pt that cannot achieve rigidity for penetration has a more severe case of ED than a pt that can penetrate his partner but experiences detumescence during intercourse.

How does the pt feel about the fact that he cannot maintain an erection during sexual activity?
If the pt is not bothered by his ED, consider not treating him.

How is the pt's libido?
Low sexual desire may be indicative of low testosterone levels.

What other medical problems does the pt have?
Other medical illnesses may cause erectile dysfunction.
- Causes of ED can be broken into vascular, neurogenic, hormonal/endocrine, psychogenic, idiopathic, and a combination of any of these factors.

Does the pt have a history of penile trauma or curvature to the penis?
Trauma to the penis can cause the development of a plaque in the tunica albuginea (Peyronie's disease).
- The penile plaque can cause curvature of the penis and prevent compression of emissary veins during an erection, which impedes the sequestering of blood in the penis to maintain an erection.

 Perform a physical exam

Perform a genitourinary exam
Assess sensation of the genitalia as you examine the pt. Assess for penile numbness. Assess the phallus and note testicular size.

Assess prostate for inflammation and induration
Prostatitis can be associated with ED.

Evaluate peripheral pulses
Feel peripheral pulses to evaluate for peripheral vascular disease.

Perform a neurologic examination
It is important to evaluate for peripheral neuropathy.

Obtain SHIM score (sexual health inventory for men) questionnaire
Scores less than 21 of a possible 25 indicate ED.

Consider nocturnal penile tumescence testing
Measure nocturnal penile tumescence with a RIGScan, stamp test, or sleep laboratory study.

Consider duplex ultrasound studies
Duplex ultrasound can be performed to evaluate blood flow to the penis.

Consider cavernosal vascular and pressure studies
Arteriography/cavernosonography and cavernosometry can be to done to further assess blood flow to and from the corpora cavernosa and cavernosal pressures.

Erectile Dysfunction

Definition
ED is the inability to maintain a satisfactory erection until orgasm is achieved. The causes of ED can be broken down into vascular, neurogenic, endocrine, psychogenic, and idiopathic causes.

Differential diagnosis
Vascular causes are from inadequate blood supply to the corpora cavernosa or from the blood exiting the corpora prematurely.
Neurogenic ED results from systemic diseases, such as diabetes, that damage the parasympathetic nerve supply to the penis.
Endocrine causes of ED include hypogonadism, hyperprolactinemia, hypothyroidism/hyperthyroidism, and liver cirrhosis.
Psychogenic causes include depression, anxiety, and failure to be aroused.

Treatment options

Consider oral therapies as first-line therapies
Correction of the hormone abnormality in pts with endocrine causes of ED may cure their ED.

- Oral type 5 phosphodiesterase inhibitors (sildenafil, tadalafil, and vardenafil) are the first-line therapy for ED in pts without hormonal abnormalities.
  - All agents have been shown to improve erectile function and pt satisfaction when compared to placebo.
  - Tadalafil has a longer half-life (18.5 hours) than vardenafil or sildenafil.
- Type 5 phosphodiesterase inhibitors work by inhibiting the breakdown of cyclic guanosine monophosphate (GMP). Cyclic GMP promotes cavernosal smooth muscle relaxation.

Consider second-line therapies
Second-line therapy includes the use of a vacuum erection device, intraurethral alprostadil, or intracavernosal alprostadil.
- Alprostadil is a prostaglandin E1 agonist that causes cavernosal smooth muscle relaxation.
- If pts fail the second-line therapies or they are uncomfortable using the second-line therapies, penile prosthesis is indicated.

When was the last time the pt was able to sustain an erection firm enough for penetration and stay firm until orgasm was achieved?
This lets the physician know when the pt began to have erectile dysfunction (ED).

Does the pt achieve nocturnal erections?
If the pt can achieve erections while asleep or awakens with an erection, then the pt has psychogenic ED.

Has the pt experienced erections with a different sexual partner?
If a pt is able to achieve and sustain erections with a different partner, then the pt has psychogenic ED.

Can the pt get firm enough to penetrate into his partner? Can he maintain rigidity until he reaches orgasm?
This helps the physician quantify how bad the pt's ED is.
- A pt that cannot achieve rigidity for penetration has a more severe case of ED than a pt that can penetrate his partner but experiences detumescence during intercourse.

How is the pt's libido?
Low sexual desire may be indicative of low testosterone levels.

Does the pt have any a history of penile trauma or curvature to the penis?
Trauma to the penis can cause the development of a plaque in the tunica albuginea (Peyronie's disease).
- The penile plaque can cause curvature of the penis and prevent compression of emissary veins during an erection, which impedes the sequestering of blood in the penis to maintain an erection.

What oral agent has the pt tried for erectile dysfunction and is the pt using the medication properly?
The physician must educate the pt and make sure that he is taking the medication properly. Sildenafil and vardenafil should be ingested on an empty stomach 1 hour before intercourse. Pts also need to be aware that stimulation is still required to achieve an erection. Some pts have the false notion that the oral agent alone will give them an erection.

Perform a physical exam

Perform a genitourinary examination
Assess sensation of the genitalia during the examination. Assess for penile numbness. Perform a digital rectal examination and evaluate the testes for masses.

Perform a vascular examination
Feel peripheral pulses to evaluate for peripheral vascular disease. Do a thorough neurologic exam to evaluate for neuropathy.

Obtain SHIM score (sexual health inventory for men) questionnaire
Scores less than 21 of a possible 25 indicate erectile dysfunction.

Consider additional testing
Measure **nocturnal penile tumescence** with a RIGScan or sleep laboratory study.
Duplex ultrasound can be performed to evaluate blood flow to the penis.
Arteriography/cavernosonography and **cavernosometry** can be performed to assess blood flow to and from the corpora cavernosa and cavernosal pressures.

Erectile dysfunction

Definition

ED is the inability to maintain a satisfactory erection until orgasm is achieved.

Consider vascular causes

Vascular causes are from inadequate blood supply to the corpora cavernosa or from the blood exiting the corpora prematurely.

Consider neurogenic causes

Neurogenic ED results from systemic diseases, such as diabetes, that damage the parasympathetic nerve supply to the penis.

Consider endocrine causes

Endocrine causes of ED include hypogonadism, hyperprolactinemia, hypothyroidism/hyperthyroidism, and liver cirrhosis.

Consider psychogenic causes

Psychogenic causes include depression, anxiety, and failure to be aroused.

 Treatment options

Consider first-line oral therapies

Oral type 5 phosphodiesterase inhibitors (PDE5) are the first-line therapy for ED in pts without hormonal abnormalities. These are sildenafil, vardenafil, and tadalafil.

- PDE5 inhibitors work by inhibiting the breakdown of cyclic GMP.
- Cyclic GMP promotes cavernosal smooth muscle relaxation.
- If a pt is not achieving erections with an oral agent, make sure he was using the agent properly and that he has tried the maximum recommended dose.

Consider second-line therapies

Second-line therapy includes the use of a vacuum erection device, intraurethral alprostadil, or intracavernosal alprostadil.

- Alprostadil is a prostaglandin E1 agonist that causes cavernosal smooth muscle relaxation.
- If pts fail the second-line therapies or they are uncomfortable using the second-line therapies, a penile prosthesis may be considered.

S **Does the pt have sexual desire?**

Female sexual dysfunction (FSD) can be related to a disorder of sexual desire.

Consider states of low testosterone.

Does the pt lack sexual arousal?

FSD can be an arousal disorder.

Common in postmenopausal pts

Does the pt have the ability to achieve orgasm?

Primary anorgasmia occurs in women who have never reached orgasm.

Secondary anorgasmia can be hormonal, psychological, postsurgical (hysterectomy), and related to pelvic pain disorders.

Does the pt have painful intercourse?

Vaginismus is a painful spasm of the outer 1/3 of the vagina usually due to history of trauma (sexual abuse).

Dyspareunia is painful intercourse and can be secondary to pelvic pain syndromes such as endometriosis, interstitial cystitis, or postmenopausal vaginal atrophy.

Does the pt have any other medical problems?

Conditions such as hypertension, diabetes mellitus, hypercholesterolemia, and obesity can be associated with FSD.

Has the pt had any prior surgery?

Hysterectomy and vaginal surgical procedures (cystocele and rectocele repair) can be associated with vaginal neural and vascular changes, which can affect sensation and lubrication.

Does the pt take any medications?

Medications can affect desire (psychoactive medications, antihypertensive medications, hormonal preparations, and H2 blockers).

Medications can affect arousal (anticholinergics, antihistamines, and psychoactive medications.

Medications can affect orgasm (antihypertensives, amphetamines, antipsychotics, benzodiazepines, selective serotonin reuptake inhibitors, and tricyclic antidepressants).

O **Perform a physical examination**

Evaluate for vulvar vestibulitis

Gentle touch to the vestibule reveals significant vulvar pain.

Evaluate for dyspareunia

Cotton swab and manual examination reveals significant vaginal pain.

Anterior vaginal wall tenderness suggests interstitial cystitis.

Examine for vaginal discharge

If STD suspected, cultures and vaginal samples should be sent.

Evaluate for pelvic prolapse

Perform a careful pelvic examination to evaluate for cystocele and rectocele. If present, should refer to a urogynecologist or urologist.

Perform screening laboratory studies
Urinalysis
- To rule out microhematuria, urinary tract infection, and elevated urine glucose, which may suggest diabetes mellitus.

Serum electrolytes and metabolic panel
- To evaluate renal insufficiency, elevated cholesterol, and liver function.

Serum testosterone for pts with low libido
- To further evaluate pts with arousal disorders

Female sexual dysfunction

Classify into a category of FSD.
Disorder of desire
Disorder of arousal
Disorder of lubrication
Disorder of pain
Disorder of orgasm

Provide education
Provide information and education (about normal anatomy, sexual function, normal changes of aging, pregnancy, and menopause).

Enhance stimulation and eliminate routine
Encourage increase of stimulation with partner education and open discussions.

Minimize dyspareunia
Female astride for control of penetration, topical lidocaine, warm baths before intercourse, and possible role for biofeedback.

Consider estrogen replacement
Estrogen replacement (topical) for pts with evidence of atrophic vaginitis and dyspareunia.

Consider hormonal supplementation
For pts with low libido states, consider dehydroepiandrosterone sulfate.

Consider treatment for interstitial cystitis
For pts with dyspareunia and voiding complaints (urinary frequency, urgency, and pelvic pain). Refer to specialist.

III
General Urology

What are the pt's presenting symptoms?

Pts with acute urinary retention commonly present with severe suprapubic pain and an inability to void.

Does the pt have a history of any premorbid voiding symptoms?
A careful history may elicit valuable information regarding the nature of the pt's retention.
Ask about previous urgency, frequency, dysuria, or incontinence.

Has the pt ever had a urethral stricture or any urologic surgical procedure performed?
Get a good idea of the pt's general health and any medical problems.

- Ask specifically about a history of any urethral strictures, episodes of urinary retention, or venereal disease.
- It is also important to ask about urologic manipulation or surgery, which may cause obstruction via clots, contractures, or overdistension of the bladder.

What medications is the pt currently taking?
Some medications may cause retention.
Common culprits include sympathomimetics, anticholinergics, antihistamines, and anesthetics.

 Perform a physical examination

Focus examination on the abdomen and perineum
Rectal exam should be performed to assess prostate size and the presence of nodules.
Palpate and percuss the abdomen to confirm the presence of a full bladder.

A **Acute Urinary Retention**

Classification

Urinary retention can be divided into two etiologies:
- Anatomic obstruction
  - Benign prostatic hyperplasia (most common)
  - Prostate cancer
  - Urethral stricture
  - Bladder neck contracture
- Functional obstruction
  - Medication side effect
  - Nociceptive retention
  - Neurologic disease
  - Psychogenic

The severity of the retention is primarily a function of time and degree of bladder distension.

Treatment is directed toward first emptying the bladder, and then dealing with the underlying cause.

P **Consider placement of a urinary catheter**

The first step in treating acute urinary retention is to attempt the passage of a Foley catheter. Adequate lubrication of the urethra and catheter is invaluable.

- If a typical 18F catheter fails, the next step is to try either a coude-tipped Foley catheter if the obstruction is believed to be at the prostate, or a smaller catheter (12F or 14F) if the retention is likely the result of a urethral stricture or bladder neck contracture.

Consider cystoscopy

The next step is to employ flexible cystoscopy to identify the obstruction, and attempt the passage of a guidewire.
- A Council tip catheter may then be placed over the guidewire.
- Filiforms and followers may also be useful in those with prior urethral surgery, transurethral resection of the prostate (TURP), or RRP.

Consider placement of a suprapubic tube

If all other modalities fail, a percutaneous suprapubic tube may be placed as a final intervention.
- Appropriate urologic follow-up should be scheduled for all pts after retention is relieved.

Monitor for post-obstructive diuresis

This refers to the excessive and prolonged polyuria following relief of urinary obstruction.
- Impairment of renal salt and water reabsorption is caused by short-term unresponsiveness to antidiuretic hormone and mineralocorticoids.
- Therapy includes monitoring blood pressure, body weight, and serum and urine electrolyte levels.
- Intravenous fluid replacement and oral fluid replacement are suggested.

Think about the next steps in management

Trial of voiding

Endoscopic surgical treatment (TURP)

Open prostatectomy

How long have the pt's symptoms lasted?
The pt must have a painful erection for at least 6 hours in the absence of sexual desire.

Does the pt have difficulty voiding?
Pts will often complain of pain and difficulty urinating, and may also present with fever.

Does the pt have a history of malignancies, sickle cell disease, or trauma?
Sickle cell disease and trait are the most common etiologies in young boys, and attacks often occur during sleep.

- Neoplastic disease may obstruct corporal outflow, and trauma may result in hematoma formation and compression of venous drainage.

Does the pt have a history of drug use or medication changes?
A thorough drug history is essential, because any drugs that affect the neurovascular or central nervous system may cause priapism.

- Common etiologic agents include psychotropics, antihypertensives, and alcohol.
- Pts who use intracavernosal injection therapy for erectile dysfunction are at an increased risk of priapism.

Perform a physical examination

Perform a genital exam. In priapism, the penis is fully firm and 60% to 100% erect. Often, the glans is flaccid. Inspect for any evidence of perineal trauma.

Perform corporal aspiration and penile blood gas analysis

This allows for differentiation between low- and high-flow priapism.

- In low-flow priapism, the aspirate is dark, and the cavernosal blood is acidotic, whereas in high-flow priapism the blood is bright red.
- Duplex ultrasound may also be used to differentiate between high- and low-flow priapism.
- CBC rules out cases of priapism due to leukemia.

Consider sickle cell disease testing in the African-American pt

Any African-American pt presenting with priapism should be tested for sickle cell disease.

Priapism

Classify according to high- vs. low-flow priapism
Priapism is classified as either low flow (ischemic) or high flow (nonischemic).
- Low-flow priapism is secondary to failure of the detumescence mechanism, the most common etiology being obstruction of venous drainage of the corpora cavernosa.
- High-flow priapism is generally a result of trauma that causes laceration or rupture of the cavernous artery within the corpora cavernosa.
- Priapism is a urologic emergency, because the risk of permanent impotence increases significantly if treatment is not started within 24 to 48 hours.

Treatment options

Treat low-flow priapism initially with corporal aspiration and irrigation
Corporal aspiration and irrigation should be performed, followed by injection of an alpha-adrenergic agonist (phenylephrine) until detumescence occurs.
- Because of the hemodynamic side effects of alpha agonists, blood pressure and pulse monitoring is mandatory in high-risk pts.
- If alpha-adrenergic therapy is unsuccessful, the next step is fistula creation between spongiosum of the glans and cavernosa using a biopsy needle (Winter procedure).
- Formal shunt creation by an open surgical procedure may be required. These are proximal shunts between the corpus spongiosum and cavernosa.

Treat sickle cell priapism initially with hydration and oxygenation
Initial management should include IV hydration and oxygenation.
- If conservative measures fail, proceed to corporal irrigation and shunting procedures.

Treat high-flow priapism with angiography and embolization
Once high-flow priapism is diagnosed, radiologic evaluation with angiography is warranted.
- Embolization at the time of angiography is considered first-line therapy.
- Observation can be considered because high-flow priapism is not an ischemic state.
- Surgical intervention may be considered in pts refractory to the previous measures.

What was the mechanism of injury?
A careful history of the event should be taken either from the pt or an eyewitness.
- Motor vehicle accidents, pedestrian struck by car, and falls are the major causes of blunt abdominal injury.
- Bicycle and all-terrain vehicle injuries also contribute. It is important to quantify the forces involved in the injury, such as speed of vehicle or height of fall.
- Falls from a height or motor vehicle crashes often imply deceleration injury.

Does the pt have hematuria or flank tenderness?
Hematuria and flank tenderness are the common findings in renal injury.
- Hematuria is the best indicator of traumatic urinary system injury; however, the degree of hematuria does not correlate well with the severity of the injury.

Where is the pt having pain?
Pain that is well localized may help to determine the extent of any associated injuries.
- Back or rib pain may represent a fracture.
- Lower rib fractures may be associated with renal injury, and suprapubic pain may be an indicator of bladder rupture.

Perform a physical exam
As with any trauma, a careful evaluation and management of airway, breathing, and circulation should be first priority.
- Then perform a secondary exam, looking for clinical indicators of urologic trauma such as flank ecchymosis, lower rib fractures, or transverse process fractures.

Perform urinalysis
Urinalysis is performed as a screening test for genitourinary trauma, although there is some controversy regarding the importance of microhematuria in blunt abdominal trauma.
- It is important to correlate the degree of hematuria with clinical suspicion of genitourinary injury before determining a treatment plan.

Obtain abdominal and pelvic CT scan
CT is the imaging of choice when evaluating for renal trauma and is sensitive for ureteral injury as well.
- In the pts with blunt trauma and no evidence of shock (systolic BP < 90 mm Hg) or other associated abdominal injuries, major renal injury is not likely, thus no imaging is required.

A Renal injury

Determine grade of injury (AAST classification)

Table 26-1   Renal Injury Grades

Grade	Injury	Injury Description
I	Contusion	Micro or gross hematuria with no renal injury on radiographic studies
	Hematoma	Subcapsular hematoma, nonexpanding and without parenchymal laceration
II	Hematoma	Perineal hematoma, nonexpanding and well contained
	Laceration	Renal cortex laceration < 1 cm in depth and without urinary extravasation
III	Laceration	Renal cortex laceration > 1 cm in depth and no urinary extravasation
IV	Laceration	Renal cortex laceration extending into collecting system
	Vascular	Renal or segmental artery or vein injury
V		Completely shattered kidney, or avulsion of renal hilum with kidney devascularization

P Treat the renal injury

Renal injuries may be managed either with observation or surgery depending on a number of factors, including severity of injury, whether there is a concomitant injury warranting laparotomy, and stability of the pt.

When surgery is warranted, the kidney is explored, and reconstruction attempted.

Consider surgical exploration and repair of the renal injury

The method of reconstruction is dictated by the degree and location of the injury. Once the kidney is exposed, hemostasis and/or vascular repair should take first priority. Any nonviable parenchyma should be excised, and there should be watertight closure of the collecting system.

Treat the ureteral injury

Ureteral injury almost always requires surgical correction.

The injured ureter must be mobilized, and re-anastomosed in a water-tight fashion.

Consider surgical exploration and repair of the ureteral injury

Treatment options for distal ureteral injuries include
- Ureteroneocystostomy
- Vesico-psoas hitch
- Transureteroureterostomy
- Boari bladder flap

More proximal ureteral injuries are usually amenable to ureteroureterostomy.

What was the mechanism of injury?

A careful history of the event should be taken either from the pt or an eyewitness.

- Motor vehicle crashes, auto–pedestrian injury, and falls are the major causes of blunt abdominal injury in children.
- Bicycle injuries, all-terrain vehicle injuries, and child abuse also contribute. It is important to quantify the forces involved in the injury, such as speed of vehicle or height of fall.
- Falls from a height or motor vehicle accidents often imply deceleration injury.

What other symptoms is the pt experiencing?
Hematuria and flank tenderness are the common findings in renal injury.

- Hematuria is the best indicator of traumatic urinary system injury; however, the degree of hematuria does not correlate well with the severity of the injury.

Where is the pt having pain?
Pain that is well localized may help to determine the extent of any associated injuries.
- Back or rib pain may represent a fracture.
- Lower rib fractures may be associated with renal injury, and suprapubic pain may be an indicator of bladder rupture.

 Perform a physical exam
As with any trauma, a careful evaluation and management of airway, breathing, and circulation should be first priority.
- Then perform a secondary exam, looking for clinical indicators of urologic trauma such as flank ecchymosis, lower rib fractures, or transverse process fractures.

- Significant urologic injury after blunt trauma is more common in children because they have proportionally larger kidneys, less perirenal fat, weaker abdominal musculature, and a smaller body surface area for the force to be distributed upon.

Perform urinalysis
Urinalysis is performed as a screening test for genitourinary trauma, although there is some controversy regarding the importance of microhematuria in blunt abdominal trauma.

- It is important to correlate the degree of hematuria with clinical suspicion of genitourinary injury before determining a treatment plan.

Obtain abdominal and pelvic CT scans
CT is the imaging study of choice when evaluating for renal trauma, and is 33% sensitive for ureteral injury as well. The most common ureteral injury in children is disruption at the ureteropelvic junction.

In contrast to adult trauma, where no imaging is necessary in the absence of shock, pediatric trauma pts should always undergo imaging. This is because in children, catecholamine output can maintain a normal blood pressure in the setting of significant blood loss (up to 50%).

Classify the grade of renal injury
Ureteral: Classification is based on location and mechanism of ureteral injury.

Table 27-1   Renal Injury Grades

Grade	Injury	Injury Description
I	Contusion	Micro or gross hematuria with no renal injury on radiographic studies
	Hematoma	Subcapsular hematoma, nonexpanding and without parenchymal laceration
II	Hematoma	Perineal hematoma, nonexpanding and well contained
	Laceration	Renal cortex laceration < 1 cm in depth and without urinary extravasation
III	Laceration	Renal cortex laceration > 1 cm in depth and no urinary extravasation
IV	Laceration	Renal cortex laceration extending into collecting system
	Vascular	Renal or segmental artery or vein injury
V		Completely shattered kidney, or avulsion of renal hilum with kidney devascularization

 Treat the renal injury
Renal injuries may be managed either with observation, or surgery, depending on a number of factors (severity of injury, whether or not there is a concomitant injury warranting laparotomy, and the stability of the pt).

Consider renal exploration based on stage of injury
When surgery is warranted, the kidney is explored, and reconstruction attempted. The method of reconstruction is dictated by the degree and location of the injury. Once the kidney is exposed, hemostasis and/or vascular repair should take first priority. Any nonviable parenchyma should be excised, and there should be watertight closure of the collecting system.

Treat the ureteral injury
Ureteral injury almost always requires surgical correction, but repair may be delayed for up to 2 weeks until the pt has stabilized from other injuries. The injured ureter must be mobilized, and tightly re-anastomosed.

Consider surgical exploration and ureteral repair
Treatment options for distal ureteral injuries include
- Ureteroneocystostomy
- Vesico-psoas hitch
- Transureteroureterostomy
- Boari bladder flap

More proximal ureteral injuries are usually amenable to ureteroureterostomy.

S

What was the mechanism of injury?
A careful history of the event should be taken either from the pt or an eyewitness.
- It is important to quantify the forces involved in the injury as high energy (gunshot wounds) or low energy (stab wounds).
- Make a note of the entry point as well as any exit wounds.

What symptoms is the pt experiencing?
Hematuria and flank tenderness are the common findings in renal injury.
- Hematuria is the best indicator of traumatic urinary system injury; however, the degree of hematuria does not correlate well with the severity of the injury.

O

Perform a physical exam

Perform primary survey
As with any trauma, a careful evaluation and management of airway, breathing, and circulation should be first priority.

Perform secondary examination
Look for clinical indicators of urologic trauma such as flank ecchymosis, lower rib fractures, or transverse process fractures. Make a note of the entry point as well as any exit wounds.

Perform urinalysis
A urinalysis should be performed as a screening test for genitourinary trauma. Penetrating injuries with any degree of hematuria should always be imaged.

Obtain abdominal and pelvic CT scan
Contrast-enhanced CT is the imaging study of choice when evaluating for renal trauma, and it is sensitive for ureteral injury as well.
- If the pt is stable with no suspected intraperitoneal injury, an abdominal CT is warranted.
- Spiral CT, while faster, is not recommended for evaluation of renal or ureteral injuries because the contrast material often does not have enough time to be excreted into the parenchyma and collecting system.

Consider retrograde urethrography
A retrograde ureterogram may be used to delineate the extent of a ureteral injury seen on CT, but is not commonly used to make a primary diagnosis. Most ureteral injuries are detected either with CT or intraoperatively.

Consider intravenous pyelography
Single-shot intravenous pyelography (IVP) should be performed if an exploratory laparotomy is performed and CT scan was not performed pre-operatively and renal injury is suspected.

Penetrating trauma to the flank and abdomen with gross hematuria
If renal injury, determine grade.

Table 28-1	Renal Injury Grades	
Grade	Injury	Injury Description
I	Contusion	Micro or gross hematuria with no renal injury on radiographic studies
	Hematoma	Subcapsular hematoma, nonexpanding and without parenchymal laceration
II	Hematoma	Perineal hematoma, nonexpanding and well contained
	Laceration	Renal cortex laceration < 1 cm in depth and without urinary extravasation
III	Laceration	Renal cortex laceration > 1 cm in depth and no urinary extravasation
IV	Laceration	Renal cortex laceration extending into collecting system
	Vascular	Renal or segmental artery or vein injury
V		Completely shattered kidney, or avulsion of renal hilum with kidney devascularization

Ureteral: Classification is based on location and mechanism of ureteral injury.

P **Treat the renal injury**

If there is an expanding, pulsatile or uncontained hematoma, or if there is an abnormal IVP, surgical exploration of the kidney is warranted.

- Some reconstructive principles for renal injuries include gaining broad exposure of the kidney, excising all nonviable parenchyma, and obtaining watertight closure of the collecting system.

Consider nonoperative management
Pts should be on strict bed rest until the urine is clear.

- Vital signs, hematocrit and hemoglobin should all be closely monitored.
- Broad spectrum antibiotics should be started.

Treat the ureteral injury
Penetrating ureteral injuries are rare, but almost always require surgical correction.

- Repair may be delayed for up to 2 weeks until the pt has stabilized from other injuries. The injured ureter must be mobilized, and re-anastomosed with a watertight closure.

Consider surgical repair and re-anastomosis
Treatment options for distal ureteral injuries include

- Ureteroneocystostomy
- Vesico-psoas hitch
- Transureteroureterostomy
- Boari bladder flap

More proximal ureteral injuries are usually amenable to ureteroureterostomy.

What was the mechanism of injury?

A careful history of the event should be taken either from the pt or an eyewitness.

- Motor vehicle accidents, pedestrian struck by car, and falls are the major causes of blunt abdominal injury in children.
- Bicycle injuries, all-terrain vehicle injuries, and child abuse also contribute. It is important to quantify the forces involved in the injury, such as speed of vehicle or height of fall.
- Falls from a height or motor vehicle accidents often imply deceleration injury.

What other symptoms is the pt experiencing?

Hematuria and flank tenderness are the common findings in renal injury.
Hematuria is the best indicator of traumatic urinary system injury; however, the degree of hematuria does not correlate well with the severity of the injury.

Where is the pt having pain?

Pain that is well localized may help to determine the extent of any associated injuries.

- Back or rib pain may represent a fracture.
- Lower rib fractures may be associated with renal injury, and suprapubic pain

When did the injury take place?

In pts with a delayed diagnosis of bladder injury, fever, absence of voiding and peritoneal irritation may be present.

 Perform a physical exam

As with any trauma, a careful evaluation and management of airway, breathing, and circulation should be first priority.

Perform secondary trauma exam

Look for clinical indicators of urologic trauma such as flank ecchymosis, lower rib fractures, or transverse process fractures.

Palpate and percuss the bladder

Palpate the bladder, and assess its volume. Carefully inspect and palpate for evidence of pelvic instability, as there is a strong association between pelvic fracture and bladder injury.

Look for blood at the urethral meatus

Pelvic fractures are a significant cause of urethral injury.

Perform retrograde urethrography

If blood is present at the meatus, retrograde urethrography (RUG) should be performed immediately. RUG is the imaging modality of choice for diagnosing urethral injury.

Obtain cystourethrogram

Cystography with plain abdominal x-ray is an accurate imaging modality for the diagnosis of bladder injury. The bladder is filled completely with 350 mL of contrast material, and then pre- and post-drainage films are obtained.

Consider CT cystogram

CT cystography is also a preferred imaging modality because of its efficiency.
Because most trauma pts will be having a pelvis CT anyway, it simply saves time.

Blunt trauma to the pelvis with blood at the urethral meatus

Determine if a bladder injury is present

Bladder contusion: Bladder injury without loss of wall continuity (no extravasation of contrast).

Intraperitoneal rupture: contrast material outlines loops of bowel, and fills cul-de-sac.

Extraperitoneal rupture: "star burst" contrast extravasation, usually below superior margin of acetabular line.

Large pelvic hematoma: "teardrop"-shaped bladder due to compression by hematoma.

Determine if a urethral injury is present

Type I: urethral stretch injury

Type II: urethral disruption proximal to the genitourinary diaphragm

Type III: urethral disruption both proximal and distal to the genitourinary diaphragm

Treat bladder extraperitoneal injury with catheter drainage

Extraperitoneal bladder rupture can usually be managed with catheter drainage only.

- Indications for surgical intervention in extraperitoneal ruptures are open pelvic fracture, perforation of the bladder by a bone fragment, and rectal perforation.

Consider surgical repair

If the pt is undergoing a laparotomy for other reasons, the bladder should be repaired.

Treat bladder intraperitoneal injuries with open surgical repair

Intraperitoneal bladder injuries require open surgical repair because they are unlikely to heal spontaneously and may cause peritonitis secondary to urinary leakage into the abdominal cavity.

Treat urethral injury when identified on the retrograde urethrograph (RUG).

If the RUG is normal, a catheter is placed. If urethral injury is demonstrated, the pt is brought to the OR for placement of a suprapubic urinary catheter, bladder exploration, and repair of bladder injuries. The injury may be repaired either endoscopically or via open surgery.

S

What is the pt's voiding history?

The most common complaint in pts with vesicovaginal fistula (VVF) is constant urinary drainage per vagina.

- VVF must be distinguished from other causes of urinary incontinence such as stress, urge, and overflow.
- Other common complaints include:
  - Recurrent cystitis
  - Vaginal fungal infections
  - Skin irritation
  - Pelvic pain

How long has the pt been experiencing her symptoms?

VVFs resulting from surgical trauma may present as soon as the Foley catheter is removed or 1 to 3 weeks later.

- Fistulas formed secondary to radiation therapy may not present for months to years following radiation.

Has the pt had recent surgery?

The most common cause of VVF in the industrialized world is injury to the bladder at the time of gynecologic surgery (75%), usually abdominal hysterectomy.

- VVF is rarely a result of obstetric trauma.
- Obstetric fistulas tend to be larger, and located distally in the bladder. These fistulas are thought to result from an unrecognized incidental cystotomy near the vaginal cuff, or as a result of tissue necrosis from a suture placed through the bladder and vaginal wall.

Does the pt have a history of cancer, inflammatory disease, or trauma?

These are all potential causes of VVFs.

Ask about weight loss, and whether or not the pt has had regular PAP smears.

- If the pt's history is positive for cancer, ask specifically about what type of therapy was used, as fistulas may result from radiation treatment.

O

Perform a physical examination

A speculum exam should be performed to attempt to locate the fistula(e), and assess their size and number.

Careful palpation for masses and lymphadenopathy should be performed to look for signs of malignancy.

Obtain urinalysis and urine culture

One must rule out the possibility of infection.

Consider a dye test

The presence of a fistula can be confirmed by instilling methylene blue dye into the bladder via the urethra, and observing for discolored vaginal drainage.

Consider cystoscopy

Cystoscopy with possible biopsy of fistula tract should be performed if malignancy is suspected.

Consider vesicoureterography (VCUG)

Small fistulas may not be seen radiographically unless bladder is filled to capacity. VCUG allows for an accurate assessment of size and location of fistulae, as well as for the presence of multiple fistulae.

Consider intravenous pyelography

Should be performed to assess for concomitant ureteral injury and/or ureterovaginal fistula.

Vesicovaginal fistula

It is important to assess the number, size, and locations of fistulae, as all of these factors will influence the treatment plan.

The impact on the pt's quality of life should also be considered when considering treatment options.

Inflammation surrounding the fistula should also be assessed, as it can affect timing of repair.

Consider the differential diagnosis

Obstetrical trauma

Difficult hysterectomy

Radiation injury

Invasive cervical carcinoma

Rule out the presence of any other fistula

Vesicointestinal fistula (intestine to bladder fistula)

Vesicoadnexal fistula (adnexa to bladder fistula)

Ureterovaginal fistula (ureter to bladder fistula)

 Consider nonsurgical management

Catheter drainage is the initial treatment of choice, as a small VVF may resolve with time.

- Antibiotics and estrogen cream are adjuvant measures to prevent infection and promote healing. Small fistulae may be fulgurated.

Consider surgical repair

Repair may be accomplished via either a transabdominal or transvaginal approach.

- The choice of approach is controversial, and no single approach is optimal for all fistulae.
- In general, the transvaginal approach is used for more distal, uncomplicated fistulae, whereas the abdominal approach is reserved for larger or complicated fistulae.
- Regardless of which approach is used, maximal urinary drainage should be used postoperatively, and pts should be followed up with a cystogram 2 to 3 weeks following repair.

S **What are the pt's symptoms?**

Common symptoms of urinary tract infection (UTI) include dysuria, urgency, and frequency.

Signs of pyelonephritis (flank pain, costovertebral angle tenderness, and fever) should also be elicited.

Has the pt previously had similar symptoms?
It is important to differentiate between first and recurrent infections, as the treatment options will differ.

When was the pt's last UTI?
Asking how long ago any previous UTIs occurred will help to differentiate between bacterial persistence and recurrence.
- Persistent infection usually occurs within weeks of a previous infection, and may represent a stone, a vesicovaginal fistula, or an anatomic anomaly.

Does the pt have any risk factors for UTI?
All of the following increase the risk of complicated UTI:

- Previous urologic instrumentation	- Urinary catheters
- Diabetes	- Sexual intercourse
- Chronic bacterial prostatitis	- Pregnancy

O **Perform a physical examination**
A gynecological exam will help to rule out any obvious sources of ascending infection or vaginitis.
- Examination may also identify the presence of prolapse (cystocele, rectocele, or enterocele)

Perform urinalysis
Urinalysis will often reveal bacteriuria, as defined by $> 10^5$ CFUs/mL (>90%), pyuria (85% to 95%), and microhematuria (50%).

Obtain urine culture
Urine cultures are ordered if the infection is recurrent, or if there are complicating factors such as a history of hydronephrosis, renal calculi, or bladder wall thickening.

A Urinary Tract Infection

Epidemiology
150 million pts diagnosed with UTI per year.

7 million cases of acute cystitis diagnosed in women/year.

During adolescence, incidence increases to 20% in young women while remaining constant in men.

50% of UTIs do not come to medical attention.

Later in life, incidence of UTI increases in both men and women.
- Risk factors in older women include bladder prolapse, gynecologic surgery
- Risk factors in older men include benign prostatic hyperplasia and bladder outlet obstruction

Mortality and morbidity of UTI are greatest in those younger than 1 year of age and in those older than age 65.

Classify urinary tract infection by site of origin
UTIs may be classified according to their site of origin, although it is sometimes difficult to differentiate infection involving the upper tracts from bacteriuria confined to the bladder. They are more commonly classified as follows:
- First infection
- Unresolved bacteriuria during therapy
- Recurrent UTI
  - Reinfection: recurrence from new organisms
  - Bacterial persistence: recurrence from the same organism within the urinary tract, despite sterilization of urine during therapy.

P Begin antibiotic therapy

A 3-day course of antibiotics has been shown to be as effective as a 7- to 14-day course in uncomplicated UTIs.

- Sulfonamides, trimethoprim-sulfamethoxazole, and nitrofurantoins are common initial choices.
- Fluoroquinolones should be reserved for resistant organisms.

Adjust the antibiotic dose for liver and renal disease
Aminoglycosides, beta-lactam antibiotics, extended spectrum penicillins, vancomycin, tetracycline, and sulfonamides need to be dose-adjusted in pts with renal insufficiency or failure.

Chloramphenicol, tetracycline, and clindamycin need to be dose-adjusted for pts with liver diseases.

Ceftriaxone, cefoperazone, ticarcillin, and piperacillin needs to be dose-adjusted for pts with renal-hepatic diseases.

Consider modification of treatment protocol if recurrent infection
For recurrent infections, urologic evaluation may be warranted. If an infectious focus can be identified, it should be removed.
- If UTIs are related to coitus, prophylaxis with Macrodantin may be effective.
- Culture sensitivities should always be used to guide choice of antibiotic.

S **What symptoms does the pt have?**

Pts most commonly present with urgency, frequency, nocturia, and suprapubic pain.
  • Some pts may additionally present with gross or microhematuria.

How long has the pt been experiencing these symptoms?
Interstitial cystitis (IC) is a chronic disease.
  • To fit the diagnostic criteria, pts must have been experiencing their symptoms
    for at least 6 months.
  • Look for a history of unexplained bladder irritability and suprapubic pain, and
    negative urine cultures.

**Has the pt had radiation therapy, changed any medications, or complained of any
weight loss or fever?**
It is important to rule out other painful bladder syndromes, such as radiation cystitis,
  cyclophosphamide cystitis, or tuberculous cystitis.

What is the severity of symptoms?
The symptoms of interstitial cystitis may range from severely debilitating to a mild
  nuisance, depending on the pt. Getting a sense of how much the pt's quality of life
  is affected will help dictate which treatment modalities to use.

Has the pt had any previous urologic workup?
Because IC remains a diagnosis of exclusion based entirely on clinical and cystoscopic
  criteria, it is important to assess what has already been done. This will avoid repeti-
  tious tests, and provide a starting point for the workup.

O **Perform an examination**
Perform a pelvic exam. A careful pelvic exam will help to rule out other pathology
  that may be responsible for the pt's symptoms.

Obtain voiding diary
The pt should be instructed to keep a careful voiding record. This will help to quantify
  the urinary frequency and urgency.

Perform urinalysis and urine culture
The findings of IC include sterile pyuria. Hematuria may also be present. Urinalysis
  can also be normal. Urine cultures in IC are typically negative.

Consider diagnostic cystoscopy
To diagnose IC, the pt should have either diffuse petechial hemorrhages after
  distension, or ulcerations (Hunner's ulcers), a rare finding. In the majority of pts,
  cystoscopy will be normal other than some sensory urgency and suprapubic
  pressure at a low volume of fluid infused into the bladder.

  • Bladder biopsy and urine cytology should be considered to rule out carcinoma,
    especially in pts with a history of smoking, hematuria or abnormal urine cytology.

Consider urodynamic evaluation
Findings are as follows: Approximately 75% complain of sensory urgency while 25%
  have detrusor instability. 20% have impaired relaxation of the external urinary
  sphincter. Maximal cystometric bladder capacity is reduced.

A

Interstitial Cystitis

Consider the etiology of this condition
The exact etiology of IC is unknown.
- Leading theories suggest a possible deficiency in the protective glycosaminoglycan (GAG) layer of the bladder, an autoimmune phenomenon, or toxic substances in the urine itself.

P

Treatment options

Consider cystoscopy and hydrodistension
Hydrodistension under anesthesia is both a diagnostic and therapeutic modality. Some pts experience symptomatic relief for as long as 9 months.

Consider intravesical treatment
Treatment involves intravesical instillation of dimethylsulfoxide or heparin.

Consider oral therapies
Medical treatment options include Elmiron (pentosan polysulfate), a synthetic GAG, and amitriptyline.
- These agents have been shown to improve urinary frequency, urinary urgency, and bladder pain in approximately 50% to 60% of pts.
- Maximum symptom relief may take 6 months with these medications.

Consider adjunctive therapy, such as transcutaneous electrical nerve stimulation (TENS) units
TENS units have been used with some success when more conservative modalities have failed. In severe cases, a referral to a pain center may be appropriate.

Consider sacral neuromodulation
Sacral neuromodulation (Interstim) has been shown to improve urinary frequency, urinary urgency, voided volume, and pelvic pain in those who have had a successful test stimulation procedure.

S **What symptoms is the pt experiencing?**

Pts with chronic prostatitis usually complain of:
- Pelvic, perineal, or low back discomfort
- Dysuria and irritative voiding
- Clear discharge and pain during or after ejaculation

Does the pt complain of fever or chills?
Fever and chills are unusual in chronic prostatitis.

How long has the pt been experiencing these symptoms?
Chronic prostatitis is distinguished from acute prostatitis by its more insidious onset.

Has the pt had a history of recurrent urinary tract infections (UTI)?
One should strongly consider a diagnosis of chronic prostatitis in men who have had recurrent UTIs in the absence of bladder catheterization.

Does the pt have any sexual complaints?
Pts with chronic prostatitis often complain of anticipatory or postejaculatory pelvic pain.

 Perform a physical examination

Perform a digital rectal examination

Digital rectal examination may reveal tenderness, hypertrophy, and edema of the prostate, but it is frequently normal.

Perform urinalysis
Urinalysis/expressed prostatic secretions: The initial 5 to 10 mL of urine (VB1) and a midstream urine specimen (VB2) should be obtained for quantitative culture.
- The pt should then stop voiding, and the prostate should be massaged.
- Any expressed prostatic secretions should be cultured and have a leukocyte count performed, as well as the subsequent 5 to 10 mL of urine.
- For the test to be interpretable, the colony count in VB2 must be less than 10^3/mL, since bladder bacteriuria prevents identification of the frequently small number of organisms from the prostate.
- Chronic prostatitis is suspected when VB3 has more than 12 leukocytes per high power field, and more than 20 leukocytes per high power field is almost diagnostic unless leukocytes were also present in VB2.

Consider obtaining cultures of the expressed prostate secretions
Cultures of urine for expressed prostatic secretions are almost always positive in chronic prostatitis.

A   **Prostatitis**

Classify prostatitis
Class I: acute bacterial prostatitis
Class II: chronic bacterial prostatitis
Class III: chronic abacterial prostatitis/chronic pelvic pain syndrome
   a. Inflammatory
   b. Noninflammatory
Class IV: asymptomatic inflammatory prostatitis

P   **Begin antibiotic therapy**

Antibiotics are the treatment of choice for chronic bacterial prostatitis.
   Trimethoprim-sulfamethoxazole and fluoroquinolones are lipid soluble and penetrate the lipid membrane of the prostate.

- Consider a 1- to 2-month course of treatment.
- Antibiotics given for 4 to 6 weeks are curative in 33% to 50% of pts. Treatment
  may be extended to 12 weeks if the pt's symptoms remain.

Add antiinflammatory medications
Antiinflammatory agents, such as ibuprofen, have been helpful in reducing symptoms
   in many pts.

Consider transurethral resection of the prostate (TURP)
Pts with prostatic calculi that are unresponsive to therapy may benefit from TURP.

Consider alternative treatment strategies
The treatments vary widely. The following may all be of benefit:
   - Nonsteroidal antiinflammatory drugs   - Hot sitz baths
   - Tricyclic antidepressants   - Anticholinergics
   - Repeated prostatic massage   - 5-alpha reductase inhibitors

Consider treatment as for interstitial cystitis
The treatment of chronic prostatitis when refractory to above may benefit from
   modalities used to treat pts with interstitial cystitis.

- Pentosan polysulfate (Elmiron) a heparinoid molecule has been shown to improve
  urinary frequency, urgency, and pelvic pain in approximately 50% of pts.
- Intravesical installations of dimethylsulfoxide have shown improvement in 40%
  to 60% of pts.
- Bladder hydrodistensions, effective treatment for interstitial cystitis, have shown
  some promise in treatment of chronic prostatitis.
- Sacral neuromodulation (Interstim) has reduced urinary frequency, urinary
  urgency, and pelvic pressure in approximately 50% of pts.

S   **What is the pt's chief complaint?**

Pts usually complain of ecchymosis and edema of their penis.

What was the pt doing when he sustained this injury?

The most common injury leading to penile fracture is sexual intercourse in the woman-on-top position. Usually the penis slips out and hits against the pubic bone or the perineum.

How long ago did this injury occur?

The physician needs to know when the injury occurred because the amount of fibrosis that occurs increases as the time from the injury increases.

Has the swelling or ecchymosis remained stable since noticing the injury or has it worsened?

This lets the physician know if the pt is continuing to leak blood from the corpora cavernosa as well as judge the severity of the injury.

Did the pt notice any abnormal sounds when the injury occurred?

Some pts will actually hear a popping sound when they fracture their penis.

Did the pt experience detumescence immediately after the injury?

Some pts will lose their erection immediately with a penile fracture while others will notice that their erection is less rigid than it was before the injury.

Has the pt noticed blood in his urine after the injury?

25% of pts with a penile fracture will have a urethral tear.

   Perform a physical examination

Examine the penis

Notice the ecchymosis and edema.

- Assess the size of any hematoma.
- Try to feel an induration in the corpora.
- Notice any blood at the urethral meatus.

Perform urinalysis

Assess for hematuria. If hematuria is present, obtain a retrograde urethrogram to rule out a urethral tear.

Consider cavernosogram

Can demonstrate exactly where contrast extravasates from the corpora cavernosa. This test is rarely necessary.

Penile Fracture

A penile fracture is a tear in the layer of tissue that immediately surrounds the corpora cavernosa, the tunica albuginea.

- This tear allows extravasation of blood from the corpora into other areas of the penis.
- The collection of extravasated blood will be contained within Buck's fascia of the penis.
- The most common injury leading to penile fractures is sexual trauma during intercourse in the woman-on-top position.
- When the penis slips out of the vagina and hits against the pubic bone, the penis bends, resulting in stretching and tearing of the tunica albuginea.
- This condition can also result from vigorous masturbation as well.
- Cases have also been reported during anal intercourse in which the penis will slip out of the anus and hit the coccygeal bone.

Consider differential diagnosis
- Penile hematoma
- Anterior urethral disruption
- Penile fracture
- Urethral contusion

Treatment

Prompt surgical exploration and repair

Immediate surgery should be performed in pts with penile fractures.

- Surgery consists of evacuating the hematoma and closing the corporal tear.
- Any concomitant urethral tear can be closed at the same time.
- Foley catheter should also be placed in pts with urethral tears.
- Delay in surgery can lead to increased penile fibrosis and erectile dysfunction in the future.

Follow-up
Refrain from future sexual activity for at least 6 weeks after surgery
Explain possible side effects of surgery such as:
- Penile numbness
- Penile shortening
- Erectile dysfunction: may require treatment with sildenafil, tadalafil, or vardenafil
- Penile curvature (Peyronie's disease)

What is the indication for catheterization? Does the pt need a catheter?

Urologist can be asked to place urinary catheters in pts that do not need catheterization.

- If the pt can void on his or her own and empty the bladder completely, then placing a catheter may be unnecessary.
- Obtain indications for catheterization from the consulting service.
- Often catheterization is performed for strict measurement of urine output.

What happened with the previous attempt at catheterization?
Obtaining the history from the person who last attempted catheterization can give insight into location and etiology of the difficulty.

How was the pt's voiding before hospitalization? Does the pt possess any lower urinary tract symptoms?
Pts with deceased force of urinary stream and lower urinary tract symptoms may have underlying pathology resulting in a difficult catheterization.

- Urethral strictures, benign prostatic hyperplasia, and bladder neck contractures all can lead to decreased force of stream and difficult catheterization.

Does the pt have any urological history? Has the pt had previous difficulty with catheterization?
Screen for histories of urethral strictures, gonococcal urethritis, prostatic enlargements, urethral false passages, urethral or prostatic surgeries.

What is the pt's surgical history?
A pt with a history of prostatectomy could have a bladder neck contracture at the vesicourethral anastomosis.

- Prior urethral reconstructions or endoscopic incisions of strictures will give clues to etiology and location of the difficult catheterizations.

What are the pt's medications?
The presence of alpha-blockers and 5-alpha reductase inhibitors on the pt's medication list may suggest benign prostatic hyperplasia (BPH).

 Perform a physical exam

Check vital signs
Fevers, tachycardia, and hypotension could be due to urinary sepsis.

Assess general appearance
Flushed skin, lethargy, and increased body temperature could suggest systemic illness such as fevers or sepsis. The urinary system may be the source for this systemic illness.
Pain and anxiety could be related to a distended bladder secondary to impaired ability to urinate.
Pain and anxiety from other sources can result in increased sympathetic tone and impaired urinary sphincteric relaxation with attempted catheterization.

Perform an abdominal exam
A distended bladder from outlet obstruction may be palpable at the suprapubic region.

Examine for costovertebral tenderness
Costovertebral angle tenderness can be present in pyelonephritis, perinephric abscesses, and stones.

Examine the genitalia

Inspect for meatal stenosis in males.

Phimosis, the inability to pull back the foreskin, can cause poor visualization of the urethra.

Obesity may lead to the inability to visualize the urethra in males and females.

Perform a digital rectal exam

Examine the prostate for enlargement or nodules. BPH and prostate cancer both can present with urinary obstruction.

Perform laboratory tests

Serum electrolytes, BUN, and creatinine screen for metabolic abnormalities. Bladder outlet obstruction can lead to elevated BUN/creatinine and post-obstructive renal failure.

CBC with differential screens for systemic illnesses that may relate to the need for catheterization.

Difficult catheterization

Multiple etiologies can result in difficult catheterizations. Some of the etiologies are meatal stenosis, urethral strictures, urethral diverticula, urethral false passages, BPH, prostate cancer, bladder neck contractures, phimosis, and obesity.

Careful visualization of the female urethra

Difficult catheterization in females results from the inability to visualize the urethra.

- Obtain sufficient help to retract abdominal pannus and genital labia if needed.
- If the urethra is still difficult to visualize, then placing a vaginal speculum into the vagina can help locate the urethra. Place the catheter above the speculum.

Assessment of the area of stricture in males

Inject the urethra with water-soluble lubricant-anesthetic. 2% lidocaine jelly is frequently used.

Gently attempt to pass a Coude catheter into the bladder. A Coude catheter is a firm catheter with a curved tip. This tip allows for manipulation beyond a large prostate. The curved tip also has a decreased chance of entering a false passage.

If failure to pass a Coude catheter occurs, then the following options exist.

- Filiform and followers
- Guide wires and ureteral catheters
- Endoscopic placement of the catheter
- Percutaneous suprapubic cystotomy

S **Does the pt notice or report any blood, or color change in their urine?**
The hematuria can be due to cystitis.

Is the pt undergoing any therapy for carcinoma of the bladder or cervix?
Radiotherapy often is a cause of urothelial dysfunction and hematuria.

Is the pt currently or has the pt recently been taking cyclophosphamide?
Hematuria is often a side effect of cyclophosphamide.

Is the pt experiencing dysuria, increased frequency, or nocturia?
The previous symptoms can all be attributed to cystitis.

O **Examine the abdomen and suprapubic area**
Look for any pain or discomfort around the area of the bladder.

Obtain laboratory tests
Urinalysis (UA) with culture and sensitivity
  • Check for gross/microscopic hematuria/leukocytes/infection
CBC with differential
  • Look for any anemia or blood loss
Abdominal/pelvic ultrasound to view bladder and kidneys

A **Hemorrhagic cystitis**
Based on previous results with hematuria-positive UA and the previously listed
  symptoms, hemorrhagic cystitis can be diagnosed.

  • It is important to investigate the pts bladder/cervical cancer history, as well as
    the pt's family history in the same areas to ascertain an accurate picture, and
    facilitate a proper diagnosis.

Differential diagnosis
Radiation cystitis
  • To the bladder
  • To the prostate (external beam or direct to the prostate [seeds])
  • To the cervix
Cyclophosphamide cystitis

P **Stop cyclophosphamide**
If the problem is being caused by cyclophosphamide, then the drug must be stopped
  immediately.
  • Two prevention strategies for the future: produce diuresis and have the pt void
    frequently.

Perform cystoscopy
Findings may include:
  • Decreased bladder capacity
  • Pale urothelium
  • Multiple areas of dilated and tortuous blood vessels
  • Bladder ulcerations
  • Vesicovaginal fistulae

Consider cystoscopic fulguration of bleeding

Cystoscopic fulguration may be used to control bleeding, but has a very low success rate.

- Formalin(3.9%) tends to have much better success. Several applications may be needed over the proceeding two or three days. The catheter is clamped for 30 minutes and the bladder is lavaged for several minutes. Multiple installations may be required.
- Irrigation with 1% alum (ammonium salt) is another option. Irrigation is undertaken through a three-way urinary catheter.

Consider silver nitrate and vasopressin

Silver nitrate and vasopressin are two alternatives that may also be applied to help relieve the bleeding, with some degree of success.

Consider transurethral balloon treatment

Transurethral placement of a balloon can be used to maintain the bladder pressure equivocal to that of normal systolic blood pressure, and left in place for several hours.

Consider inducing diuresis

Some pts respond to diuretics and frequent voiding.

This will reduce the concentration of cyclophosphamide in the bladder and can improve hematuria.

Consider catheter embolization of the iliac artery

Described as an alternate therapy (1982) and is indicated when previous measures have failed.

IV
Infertility

S **What is the pt's fertility history?**

Does the male have normal erections/anatomy?
A history of Peyronie's disease or hypospadias can adversely affect fertility.

Does the male ejaculate semen into the vagina?
This pt may have anejaculation or retrograde ejaculation.

How often is the couple having intercourse and during what time of the menstrual cycle?
The couple should realize that ovulation occurs midway during the cycle and fertilization can only occur at this time. The current recommendation is to perform sexual intercourse every 2 days during this time.

How often is the male partner masturbating?
Masturbation (or intercourse) that is too frequent can lead to decreased sperm reserves and reduce the number of sperm deposited into the vagina.

What is the nature of the man's ejaculate? Does the male partner ejaculate? Is the volume of ejaculate reduced?
The normal ejaculate volume is 2 to 6 mL.

If there is either absent or low volume ejaculate, suspicion should be raised for retrograde ejaculation, hypogonadism, ejaculatory duct obstruction, or absence of the vas deferens.

Does the semen liquefy shortly after ejaculation?
This is essential for fertilization. The prostatic component of the semen is responsible for this. Absence of liquefaction suggests prostatic dysfunction.

O **Perform a physical exam**

Observe the pt's general body habitus
Disproportionately long extremities, gynecomastia, or female escutcheon should signal the possibility of an endocrine or congenital disorder.

Examine the lower abdomen and genitals
The genital exam should be performed in a warm room to allow for relaxation of the cremaster muscle.
- Examine the penis for hypospadias, chordee, condylomata, or urethral discharge.
- Scrotal contents should then be palpated:
  - The testes should be palpated for consistency, size, and any abnormal masses.
  - The epididymis is found posterolateral to the testis. If it is prominent or indurated, obstruction should be considered. Palpation of discrete cysts does not typically imply obstruction.
  - The vas deferens is found posteromedial to the testis. It should be palpable bilaterally. Absence of this structure suggests mutation of the *CFTR* gene.
  - Palpate the spermatic cord for varicocele (dilation of the venous plexus of veins in the cord). During the exam, the pt should be asked to perform the Valsalva maneuver.
- Rectal exam should be performed to evaluate the prostate. Tenderness suggests prostatitis.

Consider a semen analysis. Evaluate semen for several parameters
Sperm count: the normal count should be greater than 20 million/mL
Motility: reported as the percent motile, normal is 50% or greater
Volume: should be at least 2 mL, if < 2 mL, consider retrograde ejaculation
pH: should be greater than 7.2
Morphology: 15% should be normal by strict criteria
Viability: 75% or more should be viable
White blood cells: less than 1 million/mL; men with > 1 million/mL should have
  semen culture.

Consider a hormone profile
Testosterone: responsible for secondary sex characteristics, produced by Leydig cells
Follicle stimulating hormone (FSH): typically regulated by negative feedback inhibition
  by the Sertoli cells. In most instances of abnormal spermatogenesis, FSH is elevated.

Male Infertility
Retrograde ejaculation

Consider the differential diagnosis
Surgical (recent urologic procedure such as transurethral resection of the prostate)
Diabetes mellitus
Stroke
Multiple sclerosis
Medication use (alpha blockers, anticholinergic agents)

Anejaculation

Consider the differential diagnosis
Anejaculation: failure to ejaculate, may be a severe form of retrograde ejaculation
Can be secondary to androgen deficiency, sympathetic denervation, bladder neck or
  prostatic surgery, or pharmacologic agents (especially alpha antagonists).

Varicocele

Determine the varicocele grade
Tortuosity and dilation of the veins in the spermatic cord, which causes abnormalities
in spermatogenesis by altering the temperature of the testis.
- Grade I: small; only palpable during Valsalva maneuver
- Grade II: moderate; palpable with the pt standing
- Grade III: large; palpable with the pt supine

Obstructive azoospermia

Consider the differential diagnosis
Obstructive azoospermia: absence of sperm in the ejaculate secondary to an obstruction. Can be caused by many etiologies including previous vasectomy, congenital
bilateral absence of the vas deferens (CBAVD), previous infection (which has
caused strictures).

Nonobstructive azoospermia

Consider the differential diagnosis

Nonobstructive azoospermia: absence of sperm in the ejaculate not secondary to an obstruction. This implies a defect in sperm production.

Multiple pathologies seen on testis biopsy, including Sertoli cell only syndrome, maturation arrest, and hypospermatogenesis.

P Retrograde ejaculation

Modify medication use when possible

For example, if the pt is taking an alpha-blocker for benign prostatic hyperplasia, this could be changed to one that can be dose-adjusted.

- Tamsulosin (Flomax) comes only in one strength
- Alfuzosin (Uroxitral) comes only in one strength
- Doxazosin (Cardura) can be dose adjusted from 1 to 8 mg
- Terazosin (Hytrin) can be dose adjusted from 1 to 10 mg

Consider medical treatment

If secondary to medical causes, the pt may benefit from medications that increase sympathetic tone such as imipramine, pseudoephedrine, and ephedrine sulfate.

Consider recovery of sperm if pt is infertile

If secondary to surgical causes, the infertility can be treated by recovery of the sperm from urine and performing intrauterine insemination (IUI). If this is the case, the urinary pH should be optimized for sperm survival.

Anejaculation

Consider androgen deficiency

Pt may benefit from androgen replacement therapy.

Consider sympathetic denervation

Pt may benefit from medications that increase sympathetic tone as in retrograde ejaculation. Two other modalities which are effective in spinal cord injury pts are vibratory stimulation and electroejaculation.

Consider previous surgery on the prostate or bladder neck

Pt may benefit from sperm retrieval and IUI.

Consider no etiology can be found

Stop pharmacologic agents that may interfere with sympathetic tone.

Varicocele

Consider surgical repair

Ligation of the varicoceles by various techniques (subinguinal, inguinal, or retroperitoneal) can be performed. All of the techniques have similar success rates in ablation of the varicoceles.

- Results in semen improvement in 70%
- Pregnancy rate is 30%
- Recurrence rate ranges from 0% to 25%, depending on approach selected
- Technical failure rate is low.

Consider embolization
Improves semen characteristics in 50% of pts with a pregnancy rate of 10% to 50%. The recurrence rate is 0% to 10%, and the technical failure rate is 10% to 15%.

Obstructive azoospermia

Consider reconstructive surgery
Consider microsurgical vasectomy reversal

Consider sperm retrieval techniques
Sperm retrieval: Seminal vesicle aspiration, epididymal sperm aspiration either microscopically or percutaneously, or testicular sperm extraction (TESE).

Nonobstructive azoospermia

Consider testicular sperm extraction
Pts with seemingly poor pathologic results can be found to have islands of normal spermatogenesis.
- These pts can sometimes be helped with open TESE.
- This sperm can then be used for intracytoplasmic sperm injection and in vitro fertilization.

V

Calculus Disease

S **Is the pt having pain?**

Renal colic and non-colic pain can originate from the kidney.

- Colic pain is caused by stretching of the collecting system or ureter.
- Noncolic pain is due to renal capsular distension.

Is the pt having severe pain?
If obstruction of renal pelvis, severe costovertebral angle (CVA) pain (dull or sharp) can occur.
Pain is constant.

Is the pt having nausea or vomiting?
Occasional anorexia, nausea, or emesis can occur.

- This can confuse this condition with biliary colic or cholelithiasis (especially with right-sided pain).
- This condition can also be confused with gastritis, acute pancreatitis, or peptic ulcer disease if pain is on left.

Is the pain worse with increased fluid intake?
Stones in a renal calyx or calyceal diverticula may cause obstruction and renal colic. Pain may be exacerbated after consumption of large amounts of fluid.

Does the pt get occasional urinary tract infections?
If no obstruction, there are few symptoms. Occasionally recurrent urinary tract infections (UTIs) are the only symptoms.

Is there a family history of kidney stones?
Positive family history of kidney stones is associated with an increased incidence of renal calculi.
Those with a family history of stones have an increased incidence of multiple and early recurrences.

  Perform a physical examination

Evaluate vital signs and general appearance
Tachycardia, diaphoresis, nausea, and CVA tenderness are common.

Palpate for abdominal masses
Abdominal mass may be present in cases of long-standing obstruction with hydronephrosis.

Evaluate for signs of sepsis
Fever, hypotension, and cutaneous vasodilation may be identified in pts with urosepsis.

Consider other disease mimics of renal colic
Abdominal tumors, abdominal aortic aneurysms, herniated lumbar disks, and pregnancy can mimic renal colic.

Percuss the urinary bladder
Urinary retention may present with pain similar to that of renal colic.

Consider the possibility of an infected stone
These stones (struvite) are composed of magnesium, ammonium, and phosphate.
These often harbor infection by urea-splitting organisms such as *Proteus, Pseudomonas, Klebsiella, Providencia, Staphylococci,* and *Mycoplasma.*

Obtain a CT scan of the abdomen and pelvis
This test is rapid, less expensive than intravenous pyelography (IVP), provides oblique views, and better anatomic details than seen on IVP.

Consider intravenous pyelography
IVP can document nephrolithiasis and upper tract anatomy. Easy to interpret and distinguishes extraosseous calcifications from urinary tract calculi.
- In an acute setting, inadequate bowel prep, associated ileus, swallowed air, and lack of available technicians may result in a less-than-ideal study.
- A delayed, planned IVP may result in a superior study.

Consider KUB and renal ultrasonography
KUB films and directed ultrasonography may be as effective as IVP. Ultrasound should be directed at areas of suspicion from KUB film. Study is operator-dependent. Edema and small calculi missed on IVP can be seen.

Consider retrograde pyelography
Retrograde pyelography delineates upper tract anatomy and localizes small or radiolucent calculi.

Consider MRI
MRI is a poor study for urinary stone disease.

Consider a nuclear renal scan
Nuclear scintigraphy can identify small stones missed on KUB. No delineation of upper tract anatomy.

Renal Pelvis Stone

Definition
Stones in the renal pelvis > 1 cm in diameter commonly obstruct the ureteropelvic junction.
Partial or complete staghorn calculi that are in the renal pelvis are not necessarily obstructive

Sequelae
If untreated, can lead to significant morbidity, including renal decompensation, infectious complications, or both.

Consider definitive treatment of the stone
Definitive treatment is stone removal.
- Percutaneous nephrolithotripsy (PCNL) is the treatment of choice for staghorn calculi.
- Surgical removal by anatrophic nephrolithotomy allows staghorn removal. Less favored treatment with the advent of PCNL.

Consider medical therapy to dissolve the stone
Dissolution of stone can be performed by acidification of the urine.
- Suby's G solution and hemiacidrin are used for acidification.

S

What is the socioeconomic and demographic status of the pt?
Renal stones are more common in affluent, industrialized countries.
Immigrants from less industrialized nations gradually increase their stone incidence.
Use of soft water does not decrease incidence of urinary stones.

Does the pt have any pain? What are the characteristics of the pain?
Renal colic: pain due to stretching of collecting system or ureter.
Abrupt in onset, may awaken pt from sleep.
- Pt moves around a lot to relieve pain.
- If stone in renal calyx, periodic pain due to intermittent obstruction.

Is gross hematuria present?
Intermittent gross hematuria or tea-colored urine from old blood is common.

Has this ever happened before?
Pts with previous stones frequently have had similar types of pain.

O

Perform a physical examination

Evaluate general disposition of the pt and vital signs
Tachycardia, diaphoresis, nausea, and costovertebral angle (CVA) tenderness are
common.
Abdominal mass may be present in cases of long-standing obstruction with
hydronephrosis.

Evaluate for signs of sepsis
Fever, hypotension, and cutaneous vasodilation may be identified in pts with urosepsis.

Consider other conditions that can mimic renal colic
- Abdominal tumors   - Abdominal aortic aneurysms
- Herniated lumbar disks   - Pregnancy

Palpate the urinary bladder
Urinary retention may present with pain similar to that of renal colic.

Small Kidney Stone

Consider the stone composition

80% to 85% of urinary stones are calcium calculi most commonly due to:
- Elevated urinary calcium   - Elevated urinary uric acid
- Elevated urinary oxalate   - Decreased urinary citrate

One third of pts undergoing metabolic evaluation will find no abnormalities.

Consider the stone location

Upper pole calyceal stones respond well to treatment with shock wave lithotripsy, ureteroscopy, or watchful waiting dependent on size of stone.

Middle pole calyceal stones respond less well to treatment with shock wave lithotripsy, ureteroscopy, or watchful waiting.

Lower pole calyceal stones respond least to the above mentioned treatments.
Percutaneous nephrolithotripsy may ultimately be required.

Consider conservative treatment of this pt

Conservative observation
- Most calculi will pass without intervention.
- Calculi that are 4 to 5 mm have a 40% to 50% chance of passing spontaneously.
- Calculi that are > 6 mm have a less than 25% chance of spontaneous passage.

Consider oral therapies to dissolve the stone

Dissolution agents
- Alkalinizing agents such as potassium bicarbonate and potassium citrate may be useful for uric acid stones.

Consider extracorporeal shock wave lithotripsy

Extracorporeal shock wave lithotripsy breaks up stones with ultrasound.
- Can be less effective for obese (>300 lbs) pts.
- Should not be used in pregnancy or with pts who have abdominal aortic aneurysms.

Consider ureteroscopic stone extraction

Ureteroscopic stone extraction is highly useful for lower ureteral calculi.
- Can remove calculi up to 8 mm in size.

Consider percutaneous nephrolithotripsy

Percutaneous nephrolithotomy is the best choice for large (>2.5 cm) stones.
- Stone removed by tract from skin to stone.

Consider open stone surgery

Open stone surgery is uncommon due to ease and success of less invasive techniques.

Suggest techniques to prevent recurrence of stones

Obtain metabolic evaluation to determine stone composition and any correctable metabolic disturbances. After this a variety of agents are available for:
- Alkalinizing the urine   - Inhibiting GI absorption of calcium
- Phosphate supplementation   - Diuretics
- Calcium supplementation   - Uric acid–lowering medications
- Urease inhibitors

S **Is the pt having pain?**

Costovertebral angle (CVA) pain radiating into bladder, vulva, or scrotum and testicle is common.

Does the pt have irritative voiding symptoms?

Urgency, frequency, and burning when stone approaches bladder due to inflammation of bladder wall.

- Often confused with torsion or epididymitis.

Is gross hematuria present?

Intermittent gross hematuria or tea-colored urine from old blood.

Has this ever happened before?

Pts with previous stones frequently have had similar types of pain in the past.

 Perform a physical examination

Evaluate the pt's general disposition

Tachycardia, diaphoresis, nausea, and CVA tenderness are common.

Abdominal mass may be present in cases of long-standing obstruction with hydronephrosis

Evaluate for signs of sepsis

Fever, hypotension, and cutaneous vasodilation may be identified in pts with urosepsis.

Consider other disease mimics of renal colic

Abdominal tumors, abdominal aortic aneurysms, herniated lumbar disks, and pregnancy can mimic renal colic.

Palpate the urinary bladder

Urinary retention may present with pain similar to that of renal colic.

Perform urinalysis

Microscopic or gross hematuria may be present.

- However, the absence does not exclude renal stone disease.
- Pyuria may be present without infection.
- Crystals may be seen.

A **Epidemiology of urolithiasis**
75% of stones contain calcium.
Remainder of stones are composed of uric acid, struvite, or cystine.
Frequency of stone disease is increasing; annual incidence is 1% in middle-age white men.
Prevalence of stone disease is 5% to 10%.
12 to 24 million Americans develop stones during their lifetime.
Lifetime risk of stone formation in white men is 20% while in white women, it is 5% to 10%.
Blacks have 1/4 to 1/3 less risk of stone formation than white men in the United States.

Distal ureteral stones

Consider the differential diagnosis

Diagnosis can be difficult because the pain can be confused with testicular torsion or epididymitis in males and menstrual pain, pelvic inflammatory disease, and ruptured ovarian cysts in women due to similar visceral pain pathways involved.

 P **Consider conservative management**
Conservative observation: most calculi will pass without intervention.
- Calculi that are 4 to 5 mm have a 40% to 50% chance of passing spontaneously.
- Calculi that are > 6 mm have a less than 25% chance of spontaneous passage.

Consider dissolving agents
Pure uric acid stones can usually be dissolved with oral alkalinization therapy.
- Potassium citrate or sodium bicarbonate are the two agents that may be used to alkalinize the urine to a pH range of 6.5 to 7.0.

Consider extracorporeal shock-wave lithotripsy
Extracorporeal shock wave lithotripsy breaks up stones with ultrasound.
- Can be less than totally effective for grossly obese (>300 lbs.)
- Should not be used in pregnancy or with pts who have abdominal aortic aneurysms.

Consider ureteroscopy
Ureteroscopic stone extraction: highly useful for lower ureteral calculi.
Can remove calculi up to 8 mm in size.

Consider percutaneous nephrolithotripsy
Percutaneous nephrolithotomy: best choice for large (>2.5 cm) stones in the renal pelvis or lower pole calices.
- This procedure is not useful for distal ureteral stones.

Consider open stone surgery
With the advent of laser lithotripsy and the newer smaller ureteroscopes, open stone surgery is rarely performed today.

Is the pt having pain?
Costovertebral angle (CVA) pain radiating into bladder, vulva, or scrotum and testicle are common complaints.

Does the pt have irritative voiding symptoms?
Urgency, frequency, and burning can occur when stone approaches bladder due to inflammation of bladder wall.
- Often confused with torsion or epididymitis.
- Intermittent gross hematuria or tea colored urine from old blood.

Is gross hematuria present?
Intermittent gross hematuria or tea-colored urine from old blood.

Has this ever happened before?
Pts with previous stones frequently have had similar types of pain in the past.

Does anyone else in the family have kidney stones? How are cystine stones inherited?
Cystine stones are inherited in an autosomal recessive fashion.
- If both parents are carriers or if one sibling has cystine stones, one has a 25% chance of being affected.

Perform a physical exam

Evaluate pt's general appearance
Tachycardia, diaphoresis, nausea, and CVA tenderness are common.

Palpate the abdomen for masses
Abdominal mass may be present in cases of long-standing obstruction with hydronephrosis.

Evaluate for signs of sepsis
Fever, hypotension, and cutaneous vasodilation may be identified in pts with urosepsis.

Consider other conditions that can mimic renal colic

- Abdominal tumors	- Abdominal aortic aneurysms
- Herniated lumbar disks	- Pregnancy can mimic renal colic

Percuss the bladder
Urinary retention may present with pain similar to that of renal colic.

Perform urinalysis
Often, urinalysis will reveal hexagonal crystals.
This finding is diagnostic of cystinuria.

Obtain a 24-hour urine study
24-hour urine study may reveal increase in urine cystine levels.
- Normal individuals secrete < 100 mg cystine/day whereas pts who get cystine stones excrete > 350 mg cystine/day.

Obtain an imaging study
Cystine stones are radiopaque, although not as opaque as most calcium stones.
- They may have a "ground glass" appearance.
- They may appear as a lucent filling defect on intravenous pyelography.

Cystinuria
Cystine stones result from an inherited defect of renal tubular absorption of cystine, ornithine, lysine, and arginine.
- Cystine stones are rare.
- Only 1% to 2% of all stone pts have cystine stones.
- Genetic defects mapped to chromosome 2p.16 and 19q13.1.
- Homozygous expression 1:20,000
- Heterozygous expression 1:2000

 Increase oral hydration
Three to four quarts of fluids/day should be ingested to decrease the urinary concentration of cystine.

Begin urine alkalinization therapy
The urine should be alkalinized because cystine is more soluble in an alkaline urine.
- If stone size grows with alkalinization therapy, drugs that bind to cystine should be given, such as D-penicillamine and alpha-mercaptopropionylglycine (alpha-MGP).

Consider the use of cystine-binding drugs
These medications are associated with significant side effects such as diarrhea, dermatitis, and mental status changes.

Consider surgical intervention
Cystine stones do not fragment well with extracorporeal shock-wave lithotripsy.
- These stones fracture nicely with ultrasonic or holmium lasers.
- Thus, most stones are treated with ureteroscopy or percutaneous nephrolithotripsy.

Consider open stone surgery
Open surgery should be avoided because there is a high rate of recurrence of these stones, which can require repeated procedures.

S   **What is the background of this pt?**

Bladder calculi can occur in males with bladder outlet obstruction.
- Children who live in underdeveloped countries are also affected.
- Calcium oxalate stones are most common in the United States.
- Uric acid stones are more common in Europe.

Does the pt have an indwelling catheter?
Bladder calculi should be considered in these pts.
- May relate to urinary stasis and infection or retained foreign body.

Is the pt male or female?
Bladder calculi is predominantly a disease of males and all nationalities.

Does the pt have gross hematuria?
Gross hematuria can be a symptom of bladder calculi disease.

Does the pt have change in their force of urinary stream?
Bladder calculi can be associated with obstructive urinary symptoms such as urinary
hesitancy, decrease in the force of stream, and intermittency.
- This may be due to stone lodging in the bladder neck.

Does the pt have any pelvic pain?
Pelvic pain can occur with bladder stones due to inflammation.
- Pain can occur across the second to fourth sacral nerves, the tip of the penis,
and the lower abdomen.

 Perform a physical examination

Examine the abdomen
Look for signs of abdominal distension.
- Percuss the bladder, which may suggest urinary retention.

Perform digital rectal examination
Assess prostate for any masses.
- Gauge prostate size.

Obtain post-void residual volume
Determine residual bladder volume. This may suggest urinary retention.

Perform urinalysis
Protein, erythrocytes, and leukocyte casts may be found in the urine.
Evidence of urinary tract infection is possible (leukocytes and nitrate positivity)

Obtain urine culture
This will establish the presence of absence of infection.

Obtain KUB x-ray
50% of calculi are visible on plain films of the abdomen.

Consider cystoscopy and cystography
All stones should be visible on cystoscopy.
Stones not visible on KUB will appear as a radiolucent filling defect on cystogram.

Bladder calculi

Epidemiology

Primarily a disease of men

Often associated with bladder outlet obstruction

Uric acid stones occur most frequently (50%).

The presence of calcium oxalate or cystine stones suggests the presence of renal calculi.

Pathophysiology

Bladder outlet obstruction causes decreased fluid intake, which leads to production
  of concentrated acidic urine.

Differential diagnosis

Primary calculi are found in children and are endemic.
   • Composition includes ammonium acid urate, calcium oxalate, or mixtures.
Secondary calculi are found in adults and are secondary to urinary stasis, infection,
  or foreign body.

Treat endemic stones by identifying the etiology and correcting it

Remove stones endoscopically if possible.

Dietary modification

Treat secondary stones by endoscopic removal

Remove stones endoscopically.
   • Consider transurethral resection of the prostate in cases of bladder outlet
     obstruction.
   • Remove foreign bodies.
Surgical techniques
   • Mechanical cystolitholapaxy with lithotrite
   • Electrohydraulic lithotripsy
   • Holmium laser ablation
   • Pneumatic lithotrite

Consider open cystolithotomy

Remove stones with an open cystolithotomy for very large calculi.
   • Consider when also planning on placement of an open suprapubic cystotomy
     tube for bladder drainage.

Consider chemodissolution

Requires a long time. Typical agents include
   • Suby's G or M solution
   • Renacidin
   • Alkaline solutions (for recurrent struvite stones)
Impractical

VI

Pediatric Urology

S **What is the age and racial background of the pt?**

The incidence of pediatric testis tumors peaks at age 2 to 4 years, then decreases until increasing again at puberty.

Testis tumors in pts of Asian and African descent are rare.

Is the mass painless or painful?

A painless scrotal mass is the most common presentation of a testicular tumor. A painful mass may derive from other etiologies such as testicular torsion.

Are any systemic signs or symptoms present?

Systemic signs and symptoms such as fatigue, fever, bleeding, and bone pain can derive from diseases such as lymphoma or leukemia. These entities can metastasize to the testis.

Are precocious puberty or intersex abnormalities present?

Precocious puberty can be seen in pts with Leydig cell tumors.
- Intersex disorders are at higher risk of gonadoblastoma.

Is there a prior history of hematologic diseases?

Leukemia and lymphoma can metastasize to the gonads.

Were the testes descended at birth?

There is a 40 times greater risk of having a germ cell tumor from undescended testes compared to descended testes.

- The incidence of germ cell tumors in cryptorchidism is 1/2550.

 Perform a physical exam

Does the mass appear to be intra- or extratesticular?

A solid intratesticular mass is suggestive of a testicular tumor, while an extratesticular mass usually is a benign condition such as a hydrocele or spermatocele.

Does the mass transilluminate?

A transilluminating mass usually represents a benign condition of the spermatic cord.

Obtain tumor markers

Alpha fetoprotein (AFP): produced in yolk sac tumors and some immature teratomas.

Beta human chorionic gonadotropin (ß-HCG): produced in embryonal carcinoma and mixed teratomas.

Tumor markers are used preoperatively and postoperatively to monitor for recurrence.

Perform testicular ultrasound

Central blood flow is absent in testicular torsion.
- Cystic components are found in teratomas or epidermoid cysts.
- Evaluate for the presence of a hydrocele.

Testicular Mass, possible tumor

Consider differential diagnosis of testicular masses

Epididymitis: Presents as a warm, erythematous, and edematous testicle with tenderness greatest overlying the epididymis.

Hydrocele: A fluid collection in the tunica vaginalis surrounding the testis.

Hernia: A defect in the abdominal wall allowing for bowel contents to pass through the inguinal canal (indirect) or through Hasselbalch's triangle (direct).

Testicular torsion: Physical findings for testicular torsion include erythema, tenderness, swelling, a high lying testicle in the transverse plane, and an absent cremasteric reflex.

Inguinal exploration and orchiectomy

Establish pathologic diagnosis

Definitive treatment plan

Treatment depends on pathology and stage.

If the diagnosis is yolk sac tumor

Stage I: Radical inguinal orchiectomy
- Follow up with tumor markers, CXR, and CT of abdomen/pelvis

Stage II: Complete orchiectomy with removal of all cord structures
- Follow up with tumor markers, CXR, and CT of abdomen/pelvis
- Retroperitoneal lymphadenopathy
- Persistent elevation of AFP and retroperitoneal adenopathy should be treated as stage III

Stage III/IV: Radical inguinal orchiectomy followed by combination chemotherapy (cisplatin, etoposide, and bleomycin)
- Follow up with tumor markers, CXR, and CT of abdomen/pelvis
- Pts with persistent elevated markers after chemotherapy or retroperitoneal adenopathy should undergo retroperitoneal lymph node biopsy at 12 weeks.

If the diagnosis is teratoma

Mature teratoma can undergo radical orchiectomy versus an enucleation of the tumor.
- Immature teratomas undergo above + recurrent tumors are treated with platinum-based chemotherapy.

If the diagnosis is Leydig cell tumor

Radical orchiectomy required

If the diagnosis is Sertoli cell tumor

Radical orchiectomy and follow-up imaging to examine the retroperitoneum.

S **Is the pt having pain and/or swelling?**

Acute scrotal pain or swelling should be considered a urologic emergency.
- Testicular torsion presents with acute scrotal pain and swelling.
- Nausea, vomiting, and ipsilateral lower quadrant abdominal pain are possible.

What is the time of onset for the symptoms?
Irreversible ischemia of the testis can begin within 4 hours.

Has this type of pain and circumstances occurred prior?
Adolescents can have intermittent torsion of the spermatic cord that presents as acute episodes of scrotal pain that resolves with spontaneous detorsion.
- If the pt's symptoms are absent at the time of examination, then one should suspect intermittent torsion and treat electively with bilateral orchidopexy.

Does the pt have fever or dysuria?
Fever and dysuria are more common in epididymitis.
- The absence of these symptoms does not rule out epididymitis.

What is the pt's age?
Testicular torsion occurs more frequently in the perinatal group and in the adolescent group (age 12 to 20 years).

What is the pt's medical history?
A past history of urinary tract infections, urethritis, urethral discharge, and urinary tract surgery increases one's risk of epididymitis.

Is the pt sexually active?
Sexual activity increases the risk of epididymitis.

 Perform a physical exam

Careful examination of the testicles and scrotum

The physical findings for testicular torsion include erythema, tenderness, swelling, a high lying testicle in the transverse plane, and an absent cremasteric reflex.

Evaluate the cremasteric reflex
The cremasteric reflex is performed by stroking the ipsilateral thigh and observing a retraction of the testicle superiorly. Reflex is diminished in cases of torsion.

Consider manual detorsion
Manual detorsion will result in immediate pain relief and descent of the testicle more inferiorly into the scrotum.

Perform urinalysis
Urinalysis and urine culture/sensitivity
Bacteriuria and pyuria place a high suspicion for epididymitis.

Consider imaging studies
Doppler ultrasound can document the presence/absence of testicular blood flow.
Radionuclide imaging can assess for testicular blood flow.

A **Acute scrotal pain**

Consider the differential diagnosis of acute scrotal pain

Epididymitis: Inflammation or infection of the epididymis. Presents as a warm, erythematous, and edematous testicle with tenderness greatest overlying the epididymis. Systemic signs and symptoms of fever and dysuria may be present.

Torsion of the testicular appendage or epididymal appendage: These appendices can undergo torsion and present similar to testicular torsion.

- If the entities cannot be differentiated from testicular torsion, then scrotal exploration should proceed.
- Torsion of the testicular or epididymal appendage may show localized tenderness to the upper pole of the epididymis or testis. The cremasteric reflex should be present. A "blue dot sign" may be present by visualizing the infarcted appendage through the scrotal skin.

Hernia: Acute inguinal/scrotal pain associated with an inguinal mass should alert one to the possibility of incarcerated and strangulated inguinal hernia.

Hydrocele: A fluid collection in the tunica vaginalis surrounding the testis. This collection may be isolated to the testis or communicate with the abdominal cavity (communicating hydrocele). This fluid collection should transilluminate.

Testicular tumor: The most common presentation is a solid, painless scrotal mass that does not transilluminate.

P **Consider manual detorsion**

Manual detorsion can be performed by twisting the medial aspect of the testicle to the anterior position and then to the lateral position. This is continued until the testicle is detorsed.

- The pt often has immediate relief of pain.
- Manual detorsion may not completely resolve the torsion and surgical exploration is still required.

Consider surgical exploration

Surgical exploration and bilateral orchiopexy:

- Scrotal exploration is performed to detorse the testis and inspect the viability of the testis.
- Necrotic testis are removed (orchiectomy) while viable testis are secured to the scrotal wall by sutures or by placing the testicle in a "dartos pouch" (a pouch made into the dartos layer of the scrotum).
- The contralateral testis is also fixed to prevent contralateral torsion.

S   **Did this newborn have any prenatal ultrasounds?**

Screening ultrasound will usually indicate prenatal hydronephrosis. The renal parenchyma is usually normal.

Does this child have vesicoureteral reflux (VUR)?

VUR can be a secondary cause of ureteropelvic junction (UPJ) obstruction and should be further evaluated with a voiding cystourethrogram.

What gender is this child?

UPJ obstruction is more common in boys than girls by the ratio of 5:2.

What other symptoms are present?

UPJ obstruction can present as failure to thrive.
Nausea and vomiting are also common.

What side is the child having pain on?

Right-sided UPJ obstruction is 2.5 times more common than left-sided UPJ obstruction.

- 15% of pts have bilateral obstructions.

   Perform a physical examination

Evaluate the abdomen

Feel for palpable abdominal masses such as a hydronephrotic, obstructed kidney, which may suggest UPJ obstruction.

Evaluate the external genitalia

Look for bilateral descended testicles in males.

Evaluate the urethral meatus

Look for phimosis. This may require circumcision in pts who have high-grade reflux.

Perform renal ultrasound

This test will reveal hydronephrosis with dilation of the renal pelvis and no dilation of the ureter.

Obtain a renal scan

Renal scan will confirm the diagnosis by showing increase in the time to excrete contrast when compared to the unaffected side.

Consider MRI or CT scan

There is no need to perform an MRI or CT scan because the previous tests provide conclusive information for obstruction.

UPJ obstruction

What is this obstruction?

It is blockage of the ureter at the level of the renal pelvis and where it joins the ureter.

Demographics

Most common congenital anomaly of the ureter.

Boys:girls ratio is 5:2

Unilateral occurs more often than bilateral (left:right by 5:2)

Bilateral obstruction occurs in 10% to 15% of cases

May occur in family members of the same family

Congenital causes

Failure of the UPJ to recanalize

Leads to ureteral narrowing and angulation of the renal pelvis

Can also be the consequence of a renal crossing vessel (20%)

Histologically associated with absence of smooth muscle fibers.

Acquired causes

Can be seen in the late follow up of vesicoureteroreflux, after cutaneous ureterostomy and after decompression of a dilated urinary tract.

Obstruction is caused by scarring and adhesions external to the UPJ, which results in fixed deformity and distortion.

Vesicoureteroreflux is associated with UPJ obstruction in 15% of pts

UPJ obstruction

Consider dismembered pyeloplasty

Dismembered pyeloplasty is the treatment of choice.

- The redundant renal pelvis is excised.
- The ureter is surgically connected to the normal renal pelvis.
- Standard surgical approaches include
  - flank
  - anterior extraperitoneal
  - posterior lumbotomy

Consider endoscopic procedures

Endoscopic procedures are not recommended as first-line treatments in children.

- Consider in treatment of the adult pt.

Is this child a boy or a girl?

Boys and girls have a similar incidence of reflux. However, a urinary tract infection (UTI) is more likely to develop in girls, because reflux is more commonly diagnosed in girls.

Has this child ever been imaged for vesicoureteral reflux (VUR)?

This is important to know because of long-term complications of VUR which include hypertension, renal scarring, and end-stage renal disease.

Does this child have any brothers or sisters?

Approximately 35% of siblings have reflux.

Nearly 75% of these siblings with reflux are asymptomatic and often do not have UTIs.

How old is this child?

The younger the child, the greater the likelihood that reflux will resolve.

• Spontaneous resolution occurs at approximately 6 years of age.

Has this child had a breakthrough UTI?

This implies that the child has a UTI while on prophylactic antibiotics.

• The incidence is that 25% to 35% with reflux have a breakthrough UTI.

Does the child have urinary incontinence?

Bladder instability is common in children with reflux and may worsen their reflux grade.

Did this child have a prenatal ultrasound?

Prenatal ultrasounds may reveal hydronephrosis.

• This may suggest urologic abnormalities such as ureteropelvic junction (UPJ) obstruction, VUR, and posterior urethral valves (PUV).

Perform a physical examination

Evaluate the abdomen

Feel for palpable abdominal masses such as a hydronephrotic, obstructed kidney, which may suggest UPJ obstruction.

Evaluate the external genitalia

Look for bilateral descended testicles in males.

Evaluate the urethral meatus

Look for phimosis. This may require circumcision in pts who have high-grade reflux.

Obtain voiding cystourethrogram (VCUG)

Voiding cystourethrogram should be performed.

A catheter is inserted into the bladder, distended with contrast material, and observed during filling and voiding.

Consider renal/bladder ultrasound

Only 25% of children with VUR have hydronephrosis. VCUG is the better test to perform.

Consider intravenous pyelography (IVP).

IVP may reveal renal scarring (blunted calyces, thin parenchyma, or global atrophy) in addition to hydronephrosis and dilation of the calyces.

Vesicoureteral Reflux

Determine grade of reflux from the VCUG

Grade I
- Contrast refluxes into the ureter, but not the renal pelvis.

Grade II
- Contrast reaches the renal pelvis, but does not distend the collecting system.

Grade III
- Collecting system is filled, but calyces are not distorted.

Grade IV
- Calyces are blunted and the ureter is dilated and tortuous.

Grade V
- Calyces are tremendously dilated, and the ureter is very tortuous.

Consider medical management of reflux

Medical management with antibiotic prophylaxis is administered to prevent UTIs.
- Trimethoprim/sulfamethoxazole, trimethoprim, or nitrofurantoin are commonly used prophylactic agents.

Consider follow-up studies

Urinalysis and culture every 4 months
- Annual renal ultrasound to assess renal growth and scarring
- VCUG every 18 months to assess grade of VUR

Consider antireflux surgery

This is indicated for high-grade reflux, reflux with breakthrough infections, noncompliance with medications, and worsening of renal function.
- Principles of surgery (ureteroneocystostomy) involve creation of an intramural ureter with good muscle backing to prevent VUR.

Consider endoscopic treatment

Endoscopic treatment with substances such as autologous fat and other polymers are currently being investigated.
- The standard of surgical therapy remains the open ureteroneocystostomy.

When does the urinary incontinence occur?

Urinary incontinence that only occurs at night is defined as nocturnal enuresis. Diurnal incontinence is urinary incontinence that occurs during both awake and sleep hours.

Does the pt have any voiding difficulties?

Enuresis associated with poor urinary stream could be caused by urinary obstruction from meatal stenosis, posterior urethral valves, impaired sphincter relaxation, or a neurologic disorder.

- Dysuria, frequency, and urgency should alert the physician to search further for associated urologic conditions.

What treatments have been performed?

Knowledge of previous treatments may direct treatment options or alert one to difficulties with pt compliance.

Does anyone in the family have a history of bedwetting?

Enuresis is inherited in an autosomal dominant pattern with varied penetrance.

Does the family wish to pursue treatments for the enuresis?

Often families seek medical advice to ensure that no abnormal pathology exists. Nocturnal enuresis may only require reassurance that nothing is wrong with the pt.

Does the pt have any significant medical history?

Screen for neurologic symptoms and diseases (example: spina bifida, myelo-meningocele, and lipoma of the spinal cord) that may contribute to enuresis. Neurologic disorders are usually associated with diurnal enuresis.

Perform a physical exam

Screen for clues for urologic abnormalities

Diurnal incontinence should alert one to search for other contributing etiologies such as bladder instability, constipation, infections, psychosocial issues, or neurologic disorders.

Examine for a palpable bladder

A palpable bladder may be a sign of urinary obstruction.

Examine for costovertebral tenderness

Tenderness could be related to stones or pyelonephritis.

Examine for lumbosacral spinal abnormalities such as hairy patches, cutaneous dimples, or bony abnormalities

The above abnormalities are associated with myelodysplasia, leading to neurogenic bladders.

Evaluate the urethral meatus

Meatal stenosis is a cause of urinary obstruction.

Reduced anal sphincter tone may be present in neurologic disorders.

Perform urinalysis

Urinalysis screens for infection and potential nephrogenic pathology.

Consider other testing

In the absence of infection, voiding dysfunction, neurologic or urologic disease, a thorough history, physical exam, and urinalysis is sufficient to diagnose and treat monosymptomatic nocturnal enuresis (MNE).

- If neurologic signs or disease is present, perform renal and bladder ultrasound.
- The renal ultrasound will access the presence of bilateral kidneys, renal shape and size, the presence of renal scarring, and the presence of hydronephrosis.
- The bladder ultrasound will access for bladder volume and bladder wall thickening, the presence of distal hydronephrosis, the presence of ureteroceles, and estimates the post-void residual.

Monosymptomatic nocturnal enuresis

MNE is bedwetting in the absence of daytime symptoms or other urological symptoms or disease.

- MNE is due to a developmental delay that resolves spontaneously with time.

Treatment for MNE

Consider reassurance and behavior modification

Should be the first line of treatment. Decreased fluid intake near bedtime.

- Bladder training increases bladder capacity by encouraging the child to progressively increase the interval between voiding until a reasonable capacity is obtained.
- Responsibility reinforcement uses reward systems to change behavior toward dryness.

Consider a urinary alarm

A form of behavior therapy that involves placing a battery-operated urine detector in the child's undergarment or bed.

- The child is awakened during wetting and then finishes voiding in the toilet.
- The urinary alarm is the most effective therapy for MNE, with an 80% cure rate.

Consider medical therapy

Medications are often used as second-line treatment for MNE.

Imipramine

Tricyclic antidepressant with 40% cure rate.

- Risks include side effects and overdose.
- Side effects: personality change, changes in sleep and appetite, gastrointestinal disturbances, and nervousness.

Desmopressin

Desmopressin is an analogue of vasopressin resulting in decreased nocturnal urine output.

- Can be given orally or intranasally.
- Results in decreased episodes of NE with complete resolution in one-third of pts.
- Side effects: nasal irritation and water intoxication with potential hyponatremic seizures.

S **Was any abnormality note of prenatal ultrasound?**

Approximately 2/3 of posterior urethral valves (PUVs) are noted on prenatal US.
- Oligohydramnios from decreased urine output can result in Potter's syndrome.
- Fetal hydronephrosis, dilated prostatic urethra, and a distended, thickened bladder may be visualized on prenatal US.

In review of the medical record, was an abdominal mass palpated at birth? Were other findings identified in this review?

Abdominal mass from a distended bladder or hydronephrosis may be identified in addition to:
- Ascites (urinary ascites from extravasation of urine from the collecting system into the retroperitoneum and then into the peritoneum)
- Respiratory distress from pulmonary hypoplasia.
- Urosepsis
- Dehydration
- Electrolyte abnormalities
- Renal insufficiency/renal failure

O **Perform a physical exam**

Check vital signs and urine output

Tachycardia with hypotension could be due to urosepsis or dehydration from high urine output.
- Urine output can be decreased due to obstruction, or urine output can be elevated secondary to impaired concentrating abilities of the kidney with fixed, high urine output.
- Oxygen saturation can be decreased with pulmonary hypoplasia.

Assess general appearance of the pt

Cyanosis and pulmonary distress results from pulmonary hypoplasia.
- Evaluate skin for signs of dehydration.
- Dysmorphic facial features and limb deformities may result from Potter's syndrome from oligohydramnios.

Evaluate for abdominal distension

Urinary ascites and abdominal masses from a distended bladder or hydronephrotic kidneys may be present.

Look for bilateral testis descent

10% of pts with PUV have cryptorchidism.

Observe voiding

Evaluate the stream for normal caliper and the presence of straining and dribbling.

Perform urinalysis

Positive nitrite and leukocyte esterase suggest infection.
- Fixed low urine specific gravity occurs with poor renal concentrating abilities.
- Elevated specific gravity is seen in the presence of dehydration.

Obtain serum electrolyte, blood urea nitrogen, and creatinine

Serum levels at birth reflect mother's serology.

The above labs assess for acidosis and overall renal function.

Perform renal/bladder ultrasound

Findings include thickened bladder wall, distended bladder, dilated prostatic urethra, hydroureter, and hydronephrosis

Obtain voiding cystourethrogram (VCUG)

VCUG helps differentiate the cause of hydronephrosis as obstruction vs. vesicoureteral reflux.

- VCUG is the best radiographic study to diagnose PUV.
- Pertinent findings include dilation of the prostatic urethra, a prominent bladder neck, bladder trabeculations from long-standing obstruction, enlarged post-void residual, and possible vesicoureteral reflux.

Posterior urethral valves

Posterior urethral valves are abnormal developing tissue that obstruct the bladder neck and result in poor urinary drainage and abnormal development of the upper and lower urinary tracts.

Place urinary catheter

Correction of dehydration and electrolyte abnormalities
Initiation of antibiotics
Urethral catheterization
Monitoring of renal function after relief of obstruction via catheter
These steps may not be required in older children with chronic obstruction.

Correct obstruction

Endoscopic valve ablation

Most common treatment

- Cystoscope is placed through the urethra or antegrade from a suprapubic tract into the bladder and then into the urethra. Next the valves are ablated by electrocautery or laser incision.

Vesicostomy

Urethral obstruction is bypassed by diverting the urine from the bladder out of the abdominal wall.

- Less frequently performed procedure used in instances of severe VUR, renal dysplasia, or failed improvement of renal function following valve ablation.

Percutaneous loop ureterostomy

The urinary obstruction is bypassed by diverting the urine from unilateral or bilateral ureters out to the skin.

- Rarely performed; used mainly in instances of unilateral hydronephrosis.

Postsurgical management

After surgical correction, PUV pts must undergo lifelong surveillance of bladder and renal function.

- Surveillance usually includes a routine pt history, physical exam, serum creatinine, renal and bladder ultrasound. VCUG and urodynamics are performed when indicated.

S How old is this child?

Wilms tumor presents between the ages of 3 and 7. The peak incidence is about 4 years of age.

Does this child have hemihypertrophy, omphalocele, and macroglossia?

Beckwith-Wiedemann syndrome is associated with visceromegaly of the adrenal cortex, kidney, liver, pancreas, and gonads.

- Wilms tumor can develop in 10% of these pts

Does the pt have any visual abnormalities?

The WAGR syndrome consists of Wilms tumor, aniridia, genitourinary abnormalities, and mental retardation.

Does the child have increasing abdominal girth?

The presence of an abdominal mass and increasing abdominal girth are the most frequent presenting signs leading to the diagnosis of Wilms tumor.

Does the child have abdominal pain?

About 1/3 of pts present with poorly localized discomfort due to acute flank pain (from hemorrhage) or vague abdominal pain.

Does the child have gross hematuria?

Gross hematuria is uncommon; however, microhematuria is present in up to 25% of cases.

Has the child had any recent trauma to the abdomen?

Often unrelated, a history of minor renal trauma is often noted.

O Perform a physical examination

Check blood pressure

Hypertension can be found in 25% to 63% of pts. Blood pressure is not usually checked in these pts. However, this association is important and requires evaluation.

Evaluate the abdomen

Feel for palpable abdominal masses such as a hydronephrotic, obstructed kidney, which may suggest ureteropelvic junction obstruction.

Evaluate the external genitalia

Look for bilateral descended testicles in males.

Obtain an intravenous pyelogram (IVP)

IVP may show nonvisualization of the kidney, suggesting complete obstruction of the collecting system, obstruction of the renal vein, or replacement of the kidney parenchyma by tumor.

- This occurs in 10% of pts with Wilms tumor.

Obtain an ultrasound

Ultrasound often reveals an abdominal mass that is solid and arising from the kidney.

- Also allows for imaging of the renal vein to assess tumor thrombus.

Consider a CT scan

CT scan allows imaging of the contralateral kidney as well as lymph nodes and the remainder of the abdominal organs (liver).

Wilms tumor
Most common childhood solid renal tumor
5% of childhood cancers.
500 new cases annually.
Peak incidence is at age 3.
Tumors are unicentric and can occur in either kidney.
5% of tumors are bilateral.

Consider the differential diagnosis of an abdominal mass

- Wilms tumor	- Multicystic dysplastic kidney
- Hydronephrosis, polycystic kidney	- Congenital mesoblastic nephroma

 Carefully stage the tumor
Stage I: tumor limited to the kidney and completely excised.
Stage II: tumor extends beyond the kidney but is completely removed.
Stage III: residual nonhematogenous tumor remains and is confined to the
  abdomen.
Stage IV: hematogenous metastases.
Stage V: bilateral renal involvement at diagnosis.

Consider treatment according to stage of the tumor
Stage I: actinomycin D + vincristine
Stage II: actinomycin D + vincristine
Stage III: actinomycin D + vincristine + doxorubicin and radiation therapy
Stage IV: actinomycin D + vincristine + doxorubicin and radiation therapy
Stage V: multimodal chemotherapy and radiation therapy

Consider modifying treatment in pts with renal and pulmonary metastasis
If feasible, radical nephrectomy should be performed.

**Remember the possibility of future development of a second metastasis after
treatment for Wilms tumor**
In 20% of pts, development of a second neoplasm is possible after radiotherapy.

How long have the child's symptoms lasted?
To be diagnosed with priapism, the pt must have a painful erection for at least 6 hours in the absence of sexual desire.

What other symptoms does the child have?
Pts will often complain of pain and difficulty urinating, and may also present with fever.

Does the child have a history of malignancies, sickle cell disease, or trauma?
Sickle cell disease and trait are the most common etiologies in boys, and attacks often occur during sleep.

- Neoplastic disease may obstruct corporal outflow, and trauma may result in hematoma formation and compression of venous drainage.

Does the child have a history of medication changes?
A thorough drug history is essential, because any drugs that affect the neurovascular or central nervous system may cause priapism.

- Common classes are psychotropics, antihypertensives, and alcohol.

  Perform a physical examination
Carefully evaluate the genitalia.

- The penis is fully firm and 60% to 100% erect, except for the glans, which will be flaccid.
- Inspect for any evidence of perineal trauma.

Obtain a penile blood gas
Corporal aspiration and blood gas determination differentiate between high-flow and low-flow priapism.

- In low-flow priapism, the aspirate is dark, and the cavernosal blood is acidotic, whereas in high-flow priapism, the blood is bright red.
- Duplex ultrasound may also be used to differentiate between high- and low-flow priapism.
- CBC rules out cases of priapism due to leukemia.

Consider testing for sickle cell disease
Any African-American pt presenting with priapism should be tested for sickle cell disease.

Priapism

Definition

Priapism is an uncommon condition of prolonged erection. No sexual desire or excitement is present.

- The disorder is idiopathic in 60%. The remaining 40% may be due to:
    - Leukemia
    - Sickle cell disease
    - Pelvic tumors or tumors
    - Penile trauma
    - Spinal cord trauma
    - Medications

Treatment options

Low-flow priapism

Priapism is classified as either low flow (ischemic) or high flow (nonischemic).

- Low-flow priapism is secondary to failure of the detumescence mechanism, the most common etiology being obstruction of venous drainage of the corpora cavernosa.

High-flow priapism

High-flow priapism is generally a result of trauma that causes laceration or rupture of the cavernous artery within the corpora cavernosa.

- Priapism is a urologic emergency, as the risk of permanent impotence increases significantly if treatment is not started within 24 to 48 hours.

Corporal aspiration and irrigation

Low-flow priapism

- Corporal aspiration and irrigation should be performed, followed by injection of an alpha-adrenergic agonist.
- This can be repeated every 5 minutes up to three times until detumescence occurs.
- Because of the hemodynamic side effects of alpha agonists, blood pressure and pulse monitoring is mandatory in high-risk pts.
- If alpha-adrenergic therapy is unsuccessful, the next step is fistula creation between spongiosum of the glans and cavernosa using a biopsy needle (Winter procedure).
- Finally, formal shunt creation may be necessary by an open surgical procedure. These are usually proximal shunts between the corpus spongiosum and cavernosa.

Consider intravenous hydration and oxygenation

Important for sickle cell priapism.

- Initial management should include IV hydration and oxygenation.
- If conservative measures fail, proceed to corporal irrigation and shunting procedures.

Consider angiography and embolization

Important for high-flow priapism.

- Once high-flow priapism is diagnosed, radiologic evaluation with angiography is warranted.
- Embolization at the time of angiography is considered first-line therapy.
- Observation is also an option because high-flow priapism is not an ischemic state.
- Surgical intervention may be used as a last resort.

Is there a history of acute/chronic scrotal swelling?

Acute or chronic swelling in the inguinal and scrotum is the most common presentation for hernias and hydroceles.

Does the pt have any associated signs or symptoms?
Inguinal or scrotal swelling associated with pain suggests the possibility of incarcerated/strangulated hernia or an acute scrotum.
- Nausea, vomiting, and anorexia suggest an acute process such as testicular torsion or incarcerated or strangulated inguinal hernia.

Does the mass or swelling change in size?
An indirect hernia can change in size if the bowel contents extrude and reduce.
- A communicating hydrocele presents with fluctuating size as fluid from the abdominal cavity enters a patent process vaginalis.
- The hydrocele tends to be smallest in the morning and increases with activity and ambulation.

 Perform a physical exam

The physical exam is the key to diagnosing scrotal, inguinal swellings and masses.

Inspect inguinoscrotal area and evaluate for hernias
First, inspect the inguinal and scrotal area.
Second, palpate to identify the location, consistency, form, and presence of tenderness or blanching. Attempt to place the index finger into the inguinal canal to detect the presence of solid/fluid structures or patent process vaginalis.

Evaluate for bilateral hernias and hydroceles
Involvement of the scrotum can be found in simple hydroceles.
- An inguinal hernia may involve only the inguinal region.
- Communicating hydroceles and large inguinal hernias can involve both inguinal and scrotal regions.

Transilluminate the scrotum
Transillumination in the absence of erythema and inflammation suggest a benign condition of the scrotum, canal, or cord.
- Transillumination can occur with fluid-filled structures, such as communicating hydroceles, simple hydroceles, and spermatoceles.
- Solid masses such as inguinal hernias, testicular tumors, sarcomas of the cord, and paratesticular tissues do not transilluminate.

Evaluate the mass for its ability to be reduced
A communicating hydrocele contains fluid that can be expressed back into the abdominal cavity. The size is noted to vary with activity and position.
An inguinal hernia can be reducible or incarcerated. Differentiating between a reducible and incarcerated hernia is imperative to providing the proper treatment.

Hernia/Hydrocele

Consider a communicating hydrocele

When the testis descends into the scrotum, a portion of the peritoneum transverses into the scrotum. This peritoneum is called the processus vaginalis. The process vaginalis usually obliterates.

- A communicating hydrocele occurs when a patent processus vaginalis accumulates fluid from the peritoneal cavity.

Consider an inguinal hernia

An indirect inguinal hernia results from passage of bowel, bladder, or omentum contents into a patent process vaginalis.

- A reducible hernia has bowel contents that can be replaced into the abdominal cavity.
- An incarcerated hernia has contents that are fixed into the hernia sac.
- A strangulated hernia refers to trapped bowel contents that have become ischemic.

Consider a simple hydrocele

A collection of fluid within the tunica vaginalis of the testis

Consider a cord hydrocele

A hydrocele of the cord occurs when the proximal and distal ends of the process vaginalis obliterate, but a middle segment remains patent surrounding a trapped fluid collection.

If the diagnosis is simple hydrocele

Consider observation

Simple hydroceles can be observed and most resolve by 2 years of age.

- Aspiration is contraindicated due to risk of infection.
- Elective surgical repair is performed via inguinal incision. The hydrocele sac is opened and inspection of the proximal cord is performed to identify the presence of a patent hernia sac.

If the diagnosis is communicating hydrocele

Consider surgical exploration

Communicating hydroceles should be explored via inguinal incision with high ligation of the hernia sac.

If the diagnosis is inguinal hernia

Consider surgical exploration

Inguinal herniorrhaphy should be performed.

- The urgency of the procedure is dictated by presenting symptoms and the presence or absence of an incarcerated or strangulated hernia.

Review x-rays that were sent with this pt. Is this a single-system or duplex-system ureterocele?

A ureterocele that occurs in a single system is called an orthotopic ureterocele.
- Ectopic ureteroceles come from and drain the upper renal segment of a duplicated system.

Is this pt a male or a female?
This is important to know because single-system ureteroceles occur mostly in boys and are rarely seen in girls.
- Ectopic ureteroceles as seen in duplicated systems are more frequently seen in girls.

Did this pt have a prenatal ultrasound?
Ureteroceles are commonly diagnosed on ultrasound.
This may present in the evaluation of hydronephrosis.

 Perform a physical examination

Evaluate the abdomen
Feel for palpable abdominal masses such as a hydronephrotic, obstructed kidney, which may suggest ureteropelvic junction obstruction.

Evaluate for a urethral mass
Ectopic ureterocele may prolapse through the urethra and present as an intralabial mass.
- May also present between the labia as a cystic mass.

Evaluate the external genitalia
Look for bilateral descended testicles in males.

Consider ultrasonography
Ultrasound is the best initial step to diagnose a ureterocele.
- Can be a follow up to an in-utero diagnosis or to evaluate a urinary tract infection.
- Can also evaluate for hydronephrosis.
- May be possible to identify the cystic mass in the distal ureter.

Consider voiding cystourethrogram
Voiding cystourethrography may identify the ureterocele and can confirm ultrasound findings.

Consider a renal scan
Renal scan will assess function of the upper urinary tracts.

Ureterocele

A ureterocele is a cystic dilation of the terminal ureter in the segment that drains into the bladder.

Location

Intravesical or ectopic

- Some portion can be located at the bladder neck or in the urethra.
- Ectopic ureteroceles are four times more common that intravesical ureteroceles.

See subsequent chart regarding location of ectopic ureteral insertion in men and women

Men

Prostatic urethra	47%
Seminal vesicle	33%
Prostatic utricle	10%
Vas deferens	5%

Women

Urethra	35%
Vestibule	34%
Vagina	25%
Cervix	5%

Consider differential diagnosis

Incontinence (stress)
Incontinence (neurogenic voiding dysfunction)
Incontinence (psychogenic)
Urethral or vaginal infection (when associated with vaginal discharge)

 Treatment of a single-system ureterocele

Consider endoscopic incision of the ureterocele as the initial step.

- If reflux occurs and the kidney is salvageable, surgical reimplantation is an option.

Treatment of an ectopic ureterocele

Endoscopic incision of the ureterocele
Upper pole nephrectomy with possible ureterectomy
Upper pole pyelo-pyelostomy for functioning kidneys
Upper pole nephrectomy with total ureterectomy and repair of the bladder

S Describe the pt's stream

Some pts with distal hypospadias may void with a straight, directable stream.

- The stream is directed downward in the more proximal hypospadias.
- A wide meatus may result in "spraying" of urine, while a small meatus can result in narrowed stream.

Was a circumcision performed at birth?
A circumcision performed at birth will decrease the varieties of procedures that can be used for correction. The foreskin is often used as part of the neourethra, the underlying protective layers, or for skin coverage.

Has the pt undergone any corrective procedures before?
The prior surgeries will affect the viability and availability of tissues for correction. When and which procedures were used should be noted. Old operative reports should be obtained to assist in the decision-making process of choosing the future operation for correction.

O Perform a physical examination

Examine the glans penis

In hypospadias, the urethral meatus is located on the ventral side of the penis, usually more proximal to glands, but can extend back to the perineum or scrotum.

Where is the urethral meatus located?
The location of the meatus will dictate which procedures can be performed.

- A distal location may allow for urination while standing and successful conception.
- A proximal location of the meatus may result in the pt urinating on his "shoes" if left at its present location.

During micturition, evaluate urinary stream
The ventral location of the urethral meatus creates a downward urine stream, compared to a distal and centrally located meatus.

Determine the degree of chordee
Chordee, which is a bending of the penile shaft, is commonly present.

Check for bilateral descended testicles
There is an increased incidence of undescended testicles in pts with hypospadias.

- The testicles must be palpated in this situation to rule out a possible intersex child.

Examine for inguinal hernias
Inguinal hernias are associated with hypospadias.

Examine the foreskin
Ventral foreskin malformation is quite common with hypospadias, and a stenotic meatus is also quite common.

Identify the urethral opening
Pts with hypospadias have their urethral meatus located on the underside of the penis, instead of the distal end of the glans.

Consider buccal smear and karyotype
Buccal smear and karyotype: determine genotypic sex of baby.

Consider cystoscopy
Cystoscopy to determine development of internal male organs is rarely required.

Consider upper urinary tract evaluation
Excretory urography can be used to rule out other congential renal anomalies.

Hypospadias

Classify according to location
Glandular
Coronal
Penile shaft
Penoscrotal
Perineal

Consider etiology
Polygenic inheritance: There have been studies linking hypospadiac fathers with the trait being expressed in their male children, and also a connection between brothers having hypospadias.

Human chorionic gonadotropin (hCG) insufficiency: In monozygotic twin births, it has been speculated that insufficient hCG production from the placenta was a factor in the urethral misdevelopment.

5-alpha reductase enzyme mutation has been indicated as a possible factor in developing male fetuses.

Estrogen exposure has been also studied as having an adverse effect on the male genital development.

Consider the age of the child
Treatment is recommended before the second year of life.

Surgical treatment goals
Straightening of the penis with chordee correction.
The urethra is brought forward to the glans penis.
The local foreskin is used to protect the neourethra.

Is there any family history of ambiguous genitalia, infertility, or unusual pubertal changes?
These are all potential markers and signs of a genetic trait in the family line.

Is there a history of early infant death in the family?
Can be indicative of a potential familial adrenogenital-insufficiency issue that has been undetected in familial medical history.

Did the mother take any drugs during the first trimester of pregnancy, perhaps not knowing that she was pregnant?
The first trimester is crucial for organ development, and exogenous chemicals can affect proper formation and organ development.

Any known family occurrence of hypospadias, cryptorchidism?
The occurrence of both in an infant is usually indicative of a possible intersex child.

Perform a physical examination

Note the size, shape, and form of the phallus

It is important to discern between a possible hypospadias and potential clitoromegaly (enlargement of the clitoris).

Look at the urethral opening with respect to size, and more importantly location in relation to the glans.
Differentiate between a hypospadias, and an enlarged clitoris with a urethra.
Look for possible fused labia that can be wrongly identified as a scrotal sac.

Examine for genital hyperpigmentation
Can be indicative of a possible adrenogenital syndrome, due to high levels of corticotropin.

Identify presence of descended testicles, to differentiate from empty labial folds
Identification of cervix and uterus on rectal exam is plausible for female identification.

Obtain laboratory studies
The following are all helpful in determining a diagnosis:
- Chromosome analysis   - Endocrine screening
- Androgen receptor levels   - Ultrasound

Four main categories of "intersex" infants

True hermaphrodite
Ovarian and testicular tissues are present.
- 46XX and mosaicism are most common.
- Can have ovary, testis, and ovotestis, or any combination of the three.

Male pseudohermaphrodite
Phenotypic male with unilateral inguinal hernia with
- Absent gonad on opposite side.
- Can be X-linked or autosomal dominant
- Androgen insensitivity
- 5-Alpha reductase deficiency

Female pseudohermaphrodite
Bilateral ovaries are present, with virilized phenotype
- Caused by congenital adrenal hyperplasia (CAH)
- Can be drug-induced during first trimester of pregnancy

Mixed gonadal dysgenesis
Bilaterally dysgenetic testes and incomplete virilization of the internal sex ducts and external genitalia.
- Unilateral streak gonad with opposing testis
- Mosaic XO/XY

Pure gonadal dysgenesis
Bilateral streak gonads appearing as ovarian stroma without oocytes
- Pt appears female, until puberty, when no pubertal changes occur and problem is noticed.
- XY present with high rate of malignancy, therefore gonadal removal is urgent upon PGD diagnosis.

Consider gender reassignment
Treatment remains highly controversial, with most agreeing on presenting parents with all the information, and allowing them to make the "final" decision.
Consult with genetic counselor, psychologist, surgeon, ob/urologist, and endocrinologist to help family determine appropriate gender placement and assignment.

Consider surgical therapy
Surgery can be used to physically "resolve" the ambiguity, but the "correct" sex needs to be determined.
- A phenotypical male or female can be created, but the issue of the body matching the brain remains to be the issue, especially post pubertal.

Consider medical therapy
Children with CAH need to be treated with glucocorticoids, to reduce corticotropin and reduce hyperproduction of androgen.

Are any hemihypertrophy or heart/muscle abnormalities associated with the child?
These three characteristics have all been associated with neuroblastoma.

Gender, ethnicity, and age of the pt?
The majority of cases are found during the first 2 1/2 years of life, in white males.

 Evaluate abdomen for masses

The presence of an abdominal nodular fixed mass, found midline can also be indicative of neuroblastoma.

Consider the possibility of metastatic disease
Possible metastatic symptoms include fever, malaise, bone mass/pain, bowel issues (constipation/diarrhea), hypertension, general failure to thrive.

Examine the abdomen for fullness/distension
Listen for complaints of fullness or stomach/abdominal distension

Obtain laboratory testing and imaging studies
CBC w/differential (anemia is a common finding)
Urinalysis with vanillylmandelic acid (VMA) and homovanillic acid (HVA) (the latter two are commonly found elevated)
Bone marrow aspiration (possible tumor cells)
CXR/KUB
CT chest/abdomen/pelvis
^{131}I-MIBG can be used for staging, as it is taken up by many tumors
ESR (look for elevation)

Neuroblastoma

Definition

Neuroblastoma is a malignant neuronal tumor, which evolves from neural crest cells, on the sympathoblastoma line.

Neuroblastoma is diagnosed predominantly in children younger than 3 years of age. Majority tend to occur in the adrenal gland, hence the elevation in VMA and HVA levels.

Stage the disease

Staging is in four categories, based on distribution and surgical resectability.

- Stage A: confined to the origin
- Stage B: extends beyond origin, but remains unilateral, possible ipsilateral lymph nodes
- Stage C: extends beyond midline, possible regional lymph node involvement (unresectable)
- Stage D: systemic spread to skeletal organs, soft tissue, and distant lymph nodes
- Stage E: A and B tumors, but including distant metastasis

Consider surgical resection

If tumor is resectable, surgery is primary treatment, followed by radiotherapy of the tumor bed.

Consider chemotherapy for advanced disease

In the case of disseminated disease, chemotherapy is primary treatment (cisplatin, doxorubicin, cyclophosphamide, and the epipodophyllotoxin).

Discuss prognosis with pt's family

Overall prognosis is poor, and chemotherapy treatment is hampered by the large number of non-proliferating cells.

5-year prognosis for children younger than 1 year of age at time of diagnosis and treatment is 75%

Little, if any progress has been made over the past 20 years, and neuroblastoma continues to be a frustrating disease to treat and manage.

S

Where, when, and by what means was the mass first located?
In the neonate, an abdominal mass is usually identified via ultrasound.
- Right or left flank mass can indicate involvement of the kidney.
- Non-retroperitoneal masses usually fall into the category of either neuroblastoma or adrenal hemorrhage.

Has the mass changed in size over the period of one week?
Minimal size change tends to be indicative of neuroblastoma.

Is the neonate able to produce urine regularly?
Ureteropelvic junction obstruction can affect urine output, and create a hydronephrotic mass in the flank abdomen.

Perform a physical examination

Assess kidneys bilaterally
Renal dysplasia can cause solitary renal hypertrophy (on the contralateral side), as a compensatory measure to supplement the non-functioning dysplastic kidney.

Assess mass characteristics
Can be an involuting neuroblastoma or a resolving adrenal hemorrhage.

Perform laboratory testing
Ultrasound (abdominal/pelvic)
CXR (rule out lung metastasis)
Urinalysis, vanillylmandelic acid/homovanillic acid (neuroblastoma)
Voiding cystourethrography (VCUG)

Neonatal abdominal mass

Consider differential diagnosis

Wilms tumor
multicystic dysplasia of the kidney
mesoblastic nephroma
intrarenal neuroblastoma
adrenal hemmorhage

 Treat neuroblastoma

Neuroblastoma: tumors can spontaneously resolve and can be documented via serial films.

♦ Surgical removal is the primary means of treatment for stage 1 and 2 neuroblastomas.

♦ Chemotherapy and radiation are preferably avoided, but in cases where staging is beyond stage 2, it is appropriate.

Treat multicystic dysplasia

The affected kidney is removed primarily due to concern for potential malignancy.

• Standard protocol requires the kidney to be followed with US annually, until the age of 5 years, or involution is seen.

Treat Wilms tumor

Post nephrectomy, the retroperitoneal lymph nodes, as well as the contralateral kidney need to be examined for proper staging.

• Radiation tends to be discouraged in neonates and children due to the possibilities of growth problems, and toxic issues concerning cardiovascular, pulmonary, and hepatic systems.

Treat mesoblastic nephroma

The origin tends to be revealed only through postoperative pathology.

• It is often unable to be differentiated from Wilms tumor, and therefore the affected kidney is removed, before its etiology is known.

Treat adrenal hemorrhage

Treatment is supportive, with serial film monitoring. As the clot resolves, ultrasound is used to monitor the decreasing size of the adrenal gland, and resolution of the obstruction.

Index